THE PEARLS SERIES®

Series Editors

Steven A. Sahn, M.D.
Professor of Medicine
Director, Division of Pulmonary
 and Critical Care Medicine
Medical University of South
 Carolina
Charleston, South Carolina

John E. Heffner, M.D.
Professor of Clinical Medicine
University of Arizona
 Health Sciences Center
Chairman, Academic Internal Medicine
St. Joseph's Hospital and Medical Center
Phoenix, Arizona

The books in The Pearls Series® contain 75–100 case presentations that provide valuable information that is not readily available in standard textbooks. The problem-oriented approach is ideal for self-study and for board review. A brief clinical vignette is presented, including physical examination and laboratory findings, accompanied by a radiograph, EKG, or other pertinent illustration. The reader is encouraged to consider a differential diagnosis and formulate a plan for diagnosis and treatment. The subsequent page discloses the diagnosis, followed by a discussion of the case, clinical pearls, and two or three key references.

CARDIOLOGY PEARLS
Blase A. Carabello, MD, William L. Ballard, MD, and **Peter C. Gazes, MD,** Medical University of South Carolina, Charleston, South Carolina
1994/233 pages/illustrated/ISBN 0-932883-96-6

CRITICAL CARE PEARLS
Steven A. Sahn, MD, Medical University of South Carolina, Charleston, South Carolina, and **John E. Heffner, MD,** St. Joseph's Hospital and Medical Center, Phoenix, Arizona
1989/300 pages/illustrated/ISBN 0-932883-24-9

INTERNAL MEDICINE PEARLS
Clay B. Marsh, MD, and **Ernest L. Mazzaferri, MD,** The Ohio State University College of Medicine, Columbus, Ohio
1992/300 pages/90 illustrations/ISBN 1-56053-024-3

PULMONARY PEARLS
Steven A. Sahn, MD, Medical University of South Carolina, Charleston, South Carolina, and **John E. Heffner, MD,** St. Joseph's Hospital and Medical Center, Phoenix, Arizona
1988/250 pages/illustrated/ISBN 0-932883-16-8

PULMONARY PEARLS II
Steven A. Sahn, MD, Medical University of South Carolina, Charleston, South Carolina, and **John E. Heffner, MD,** St. Joseph's Hospital and Medical Center, Phoenix, Arizona
1995/300 pages/illustrated/ISBN 1-56053-121-5

RHEUMATOLOGY PEARLS
Richard M. Silver, MD, and **Edwin A. Smith, MD,** Medical University of South Carolina, Charleston, South Carolina
1997/192 pages/illustrated/ISBN 1-56053-201-7

TUBERCULOSIS PEARLS
Neil W. Schluger, MD, and **Timothy J. Harkin, MD,** Bellevue Hospital and NYU Medical Center, New York, New York
1996/220 pages/illustrated/ISBN 1-56053-156-8

CONTENTS

EDITORS' FOREWORD

In all ages, physicians have delighted in solving challenging clinical problems. Not only do patients benefit from a well-directed diagnostic approach, but clinicians experience a unique sense of professional satisfaction when years of experience pry open a diagnostic dilemma.

The Pearls Series® is directed toward this aspect of the physician's nature. In editing these books, we have attempted to develop a consistent format and style that challenge the reader with the salient features of a clinical problem and direct attention to an important question in management. The discussion that follows first reviews the patient's general disorder and then focuses on the unique aspects of the presented patient's condition. Throughout the discussion, aspects of diagnosis and care that are especially important, "cutting edge," or not widely recognized are captured and listed at the end of the text as "Clinical Pearls." Finally, so as not to lose sight of our interest in the individual patient, the discussion closes with the clinical outcome of the patient at hand. In the process, student readers beginning their medical careers, residents in training, and experienced clinicians honing their skills will find something of value in each of the patient presentations.

To these ends, we greatly appreciate the efforts of Drs. Richard Silver and Edwin Smith who add *Rheumatology Pearls* as the seventh book in the Pearls Series®. As internationally recognized experts in rheumatology, they aptly demonstrate why rheumatologic disorders are ideal topics for a Pearls book. These conditions present vexing diagnostic and therapeutic challenges because they potentially affect any combination of organ systems and encompass a wide spectrum of pathophysiologic mechanisms. Consequently, rheumatologists are frequently called upon to provide a unifying diagnosis when peculiar and seemingly unrelated clinical findings stump other clinicians. Drs. Silver and Smith demonstrate in the case presentations that follow how mastery of "Clinical Pearls" can provide the keys for resolving these difficult clinical problems.

John E. Heffner, M.D.
Steven A. Sahn, M.D.
Editors, The Pearls Series®

PREFACE

Rheumatology Pearls is the latest volume in The Pearls Series® edited by Drs. Steven Sahn and John Heffner. This book is a compilation of interesting and challenging cases seen at the Medical University of South Carolina over the past decade. Each case is unique and illustrates one or more diagnostic or therapeutic issues confronting the clinician. We hope that these cases will challenge the reader to consider the breadth and depth of clinical rheumatology. Cases were selected that depict rheumatic manifestations of systemic diseases or systemic manifestations of rheumatic diseases.

We are indebted to the patients, students, housestaff and fellows for the many ways they have challenged our intellectual curiosity over the years. We dedicate this book to them and to our loving and supportive families (Dunlap and Kate, Bets, Erin, Evan and Emmett).

ACKNOWLEDGMENTS

We wish to acknowledge Vicki Kivett for her excellent preparation of the manuscript and Jim Nicholson for this enthusiasm and expertise in the digital reproduction of the illustrations.

Richard M. Silver, M.D.
Edwin A. Smith, M.D.

PATIENT 1

A 64-year-old woman with dyspnea and Raynaud's phenomenon

A 64-year-old woman presented with a 3-month history of dyspnea on exertion that had progressed to dyspnea at rest. The patient had a 20-year history of Raynaud's phenomenon with blanching of the fingertips on cold exposure and calcium deposits in the soft tissue of her fingers. She also complained of heartburn due to documented esophageal dysmotility and gastroesophageal reflux. The patient had chorea at age 7 in association with rheumatic fever, but denied known cardiac valvular disease.

Physical Examination: Temperature 97.8°; pulse 100; respirations 24; blood pressure 140/90. Skin: numerous telangiectasias, sclerodactyly with subcutaneous calcinosis and digital pitted scars, normal skin over the proximal extremities and trunk. Neck: large venous A wave, normal carotid upstroke. Chest: normal. Cardiac: fixed splitting of S_2 with loud pulmonic component, grade III/VI systolic ejection murmur at left sternal border. Peripheral pulses: normal. Extremities: 2+ pretibial edema.

Laboratory Findings: WBC 9,300/μL; Hct 51.9%; platelet count 197,000/μL. ANA: positive 1:1280 with centromere pattern. Chest radiograph: cardiomegaly with clear lung fields. PFTs: FVC 2.04 L (78% predicted); FEV1 1.74 L (89% predicted); DL_{CO} 7.25 ml/min/mmHg (38% predicted). Echocardiogram: normal left ventricular wall motion and ejection fraction greater than 60%; normal cardiac valves; small pericardial effusion; dilated right ventricle with flattened interventricular septum consistent with pressure overload. Doppler flow study: tricuspid regurgitation with an estimated peak right ventricular systolic pressure of 77 mmHg.

Course: The patient experienced syncope while at home and died. Postmortem examination of the lungs was performed (see Figure).

Questions: What is the diagnosis and what was the cause of the patient's dyspnea?

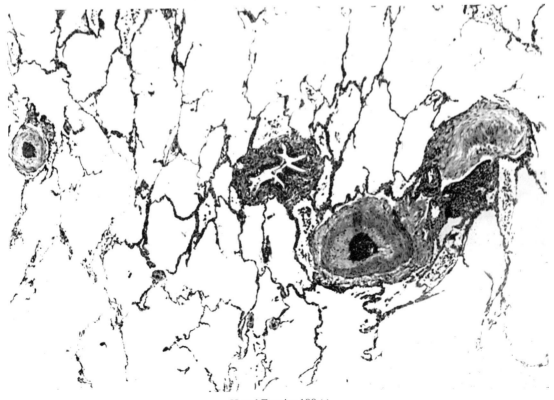

H and E stain; 100 × .

Diagnosis: Limited cutaneous systemic sclerosis (CREST syndrome) with pulmonary hypertension.

Discussion: The two major pulmonary complications of systemic sclerosis (scleroderma) are interstitial fibrosis and pulmonary vascular hypertension. Pulmonary hypertension may result as a secondary expression of severe interstitial fibrosis or scleroderma cardiac disease. Alternatively, pulmonary hypertension may occur as a primary manifestation of the disease in the absence of pulmonary interstitial or cardiac involvement (see Figure). Pulmonary hypertension occurring in the absence of interstitial fibrosis is unique to the subset of limited cutaneous systemic sclerosis. The latter is also known as the **CREST** variant of scleroderma, an acronym standing for **C**alcinosis, **R**aynaud's phenomenon, **E**sophageal dysmotility, **S**clerodactyly, and **T**elangiectasias.

Raynaud's phenomenon is usually the initial symptom of patients with CREST syndrome. The time from the onset of Raynaud's phenomenon to the clinical expression of pulmonary hypertension may be as long as 40 years. CREST patients with pulmonary hypertension have a significantly lower diffusing capacity for carbon monoxide (DL_{CO}) than CREST patients without pulmonary hypertension. Echocardiography with Doppler flow study is the best noninvasive method of detecting the presence of pulmonary hypertension.

The anticentromere staining pattern present on antinuclear antibody testing is highly specific for the CREST variant of scleroderma. Unfortunately, it does not appear to predict which of the 10% of CREST syndrome patients will develop pulmonary hypertension.

CREST patients with pulmonary hypertension have a poor prognosis. Cumulative 5-year survival after diagnosis of pulmonary hypertension is less than 10% compared to 80% in CREST patients without pulmonary hypertension. Treatment with vasodilators is warranted. Calcium-channel blocking agents are generally the most effective, yet morbidity and mortality remain high.

This patient had each of the features of the CREST syndrome and a positive anticentromere antibody staining pattern. Her spirometry was essentially normal, but the DL_{CO} was markedly reduced, consistent with severe pulmonary vascular disease. Postmortem pulmonary observations (see Figure) included normal lung interstitium with severe intimal hyperplasia and narrowing of the arterial lumen.

Clinical Pearls

1. The presence of a low DL_{CO} and normal lung volumes in a patient with the CREST variant of scleroderma suggests pulmonary hypertension.

2. Echocardiography with Doppler flow study is a useful, noninvasive means of estimating right ventricular pressure and should be performed on any CREST patient with a complaint of dyspnea.

3. Anticentromere antibodies are relatively specific for the CREST syndrome but do not distinguish the 10% who will develop pulmonary hypertension from those who will not.

REFERENCES

1. Silver RM. Pulmonary hypertension secondary to systemic sclerosis (scleroderma). In Weir EK, Archer SL, Reeves JT (eds). The Diagnosis and Treatment of Pulmonary Hypertension. Mount Kisco, NY, Futura, 1992, pp 191–207.
2. Steen VD, Graham G, Conte C, et al. Isolated diffusing capacity reduction in systemic sclerosis. Arthritis Rheum 1992; 35:765–770.
3. Murata I, Yanagawa T, Kihara H, et al. Evaluation of cardiac abnormalities in patients with systemic sclerosis by echocardiography and Doppler. Am J Noninvas Cardiol 1993;7:346–352.

PATIENT 2

A 42-year-old man with intermittent leg claudication and a femoral artery aneurysm

A 42-year-old man presented with a 6-week history of intermittent claudication of both legs. He also noted a pulsatile lump in his left inguinal area. The patient had been well until 2 years prior, when he developed a "septic" left hip that was managed with open drainage and a prolonged course of antibiotics; all synovial fluid cultures were negative. He had a remote history of a sexually transmitted disease, noted occasional superficial ulcerations in his mouth and "sores" on his scrotum, and reported a recent 10-pound weight loss. There was no history of smoking or illicit drug abuse.

Physical Examination: Vital signs: normal. Eyes: vitreous cells noted by slit lamp examination. Genitalia: superficial scrotal ulcer. Vascular: 8 cm × 10 cm, pulsatile mass over the left femoral artery; no palpable pulses, but preserved flow by Doppler probe of the popliteal, dorsalis pedis, and posterior tibial arteries.

Laboratory Findings: WBC 7,100 cells/μL with 70% neutrophils, 22% lymphocytes, and 8% monocytes; Hct 33%; platelets 375,000/μL; ESR (Westergren) 115 mm/hr. Urinalysis: protein-negative, 10–14 RBC/hpf, 3–4 WBC/hpf. Creatinine: 1.1 mg/dL. ANA RF, VDRL, HIV, hepatitis B and C antibodies: all negative. SPEP: polyclonal elevation of gamma globulins. C3: 196 mg/dL (normal); C4: 26.8 mg/dL (normal). Nerve conduction studies: normal. Arteriogram of left femoral artery: see Figure.

Question: What is the diagnosis?

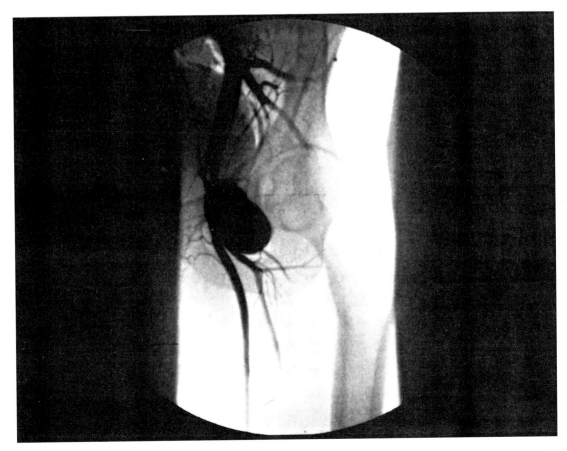

Diagnosis: Behçet's syndrome.

Discussion: Behçet's syndrome is a systemic vasculitis that occurs most commonly in patients from Mediterranean regions, the Middle East, and the Far East. Interestingly, the highest prevalences are in Turkey, Iran, and Japan, all of which lie along the old silk route. Although the etiology of this condition is unknown, Behçet's syndrome is associated with HLA antigen B51, which confers a relative risk of 5 to 10 compared with individuals who do not have this haplotype.

Behçet's syndrome is primarily characterized by recurrent aphthous ulcerations of the oral mucosa and genitalia (scrotum, penile shaft, glans, labia, vagina, or cervix). Rashes may take the form of folliculitis or erythema nodosum. An especially unique aspect of the disease is termed "pathergy"—a condition wherein papules or pustules develop at the site of a cutaneous needlestick. Visceral involvement, however, represents the more serious clinical aspect of the disease. Patients may develop posterior and anterior uveitis, nonerosive oligoarthritis, superficial thrombophlebitis, deep venous thrombosis, meningoencephalitis with cranial nerve, cortical, and cerebellar involvement, and complications involving the venous and arterial circulation.

Venous complications of Behçet's syndrome include both superficial and deep venous thrombosis. Patients with deep venous thrombosis may develop pulmonary thromboembolism. Aneurysmal dilatations, which are rare but life-threatening complications, represent the major arterial lesions of Behçet's syndrome. Aneurysms can develop within any segment of the aorta as well as in the carotid, subclavian, femoral, popliteal, or pulmonary arteries. Associated clinical conditions vary and include claudication, stroke, gangrene, systemic hypertension, abdominal angina, hemoptysis, and aortic rupture.

When patients present with aneurysms of medium- to large-sized vessels, the differential diagnosis, in addition to Behçet's syndrome, includes other systemic vasculitides and mycotic aneurysms. Mycotic aneurysms require a careful search for an intravascular site of infection, such as endocarditis, with blood cultures and echocardiographic studies. Polyarteritis nodosa (PAN) also should be considered, as this condition affects medium-sized arteries; however, it rarely produces aneurysms of the size noted in the present patient. Large vessels may be affected by the giant cell arteritides, temporal arteritis, or Takayasu's arteritis, but these conditions typically produce stenotic rather than aneurysmal lesions that usually are limited to the aortic arch branches.

The diagnosis of Behçet's syndrome is made clinically and requires a history of recurrent oral aphthous ulcers and two of the following: genital ulceration, uveitis or retinal vasculitis, cutaneous pustules or erythema nodosum, large vessel vasculitis, or meningoencephalitis.

Treatment of Behçet's syndrome requires high-dose oral glucocorticoids and other immunosuppressive agents to control the clinical manifestations of the disease. Commonly used immunosuppressives include chlorambucil, azathioprine, and cyclosporine A. Treatment is successful in 70% to 80% of patients and is continued for at least 1 year after the onset of clinical remission. Relapses occur in up to 25% of patients after treatment is discontinued, requiring reinstitution of therapy.

The present patient had typical manifestations of Behçet's syndrome with oral aphthous ulcerations, genital ulcerations, uveitis, and arteriographic evidence of a femoral artery aneurysm. It is likely that the "septic" hip treated 2 years previously was a manifestation of vasculitis not appreciated at that time. Treatment with prednisone, 60 mg/day, and azathioprine, 100 mg/day, was effective. The prednisone was tapered and discontinued after 1 year, and he remains in remission on azathioprine.

Clinical Pearls

1. Behçet's syndrome is a systemic vasculitis notable for recurrent oral and genital ulcerations.

2. Behçet's syndrome is most commonly found in the Mediterranean area, Turkey, and Japan, all located along the old "silk trade route." Although this has led to speculation of an infectious cause, the etiology of Behçet's syndrome remains unknown.

3. In contrast to the arterial stenoses associated with giant cell arteritis, patients with Behçet's syndrome develop aneurysmal dilatations of medium- to large-size vessels in diverse regions of the body.

4. An especially unique aspect of Behçet's syndrome is "pathergy," a condition where papules or pustules develop at sites of cutaneous needlesticks.

REFERENCES

1. O'Duffy JD, Robertson DM, Goldstein NP. Chlorambucil in the treatment of uveitis and meningoencephalitis of Behçet's disease. Am J Med 1984;76:75–84.
2. O'Duffy JD. Vasculitis in Behçet's disease. Rheum Dis Clin North Am 1990;16:423–431.
3. Yazici H, Pazarli H, Barnes CG, et al. A controlled trial of azathioprine in Behçet's disease. N Engl J Med 1990;322:281–285.

PATIENT 3

A 42-year-old man with red eyes and ears

A 42-year-old man presented with a 1-year history of painful and swollen red ears accompanied by redness of both eyes and diminished hearing. He also complained of painful, swollen hands that interfered with his ability to work as a mechanic. The patient denied other joint complaints and had no history of vertigo, decreased visual acuity, dyspnea, stridor, or hoarseness.

Physical Examination: Temperature 98.9°; pulse 68; respirations 18; blood pressure 120/80. Skin: normal. HEENT: Moderate scleral injection bilaterally on normal fundoscopic examination and visual acuity of 20/20 OD and 20/25 OS; tender auricular swelling with dusky erythema and obliteration of the antihelix (see Figure); the diameter of each external os was one-third of normal size; mild conductive hearing loss; nontender nasal septal cartilage and normal oral mucosa. Neck: midline trachea without tenderness. Chest: normal. Cardiac: normal. Neurologic: normal. Musculoskeletal: full range of motion without synovitis.

Laboratory Findings: WBC 11,200/μL; Hct 46.0%; platelet count 282,000/μL; ESR 7mm/hr; serum chemistries normal; urinalysis normal; creatinine clearance 156 ml/min; ANA negative; RF negative. Chest radiograph: normal. PFTs: normal. Echocardiogram: normal.

Course: Treatment with an oral nonsteroidal anti-inflammatory agent and steroid eye drops resulted in prompt improvement in the ocular erythema and arthralgia but no change in the auricular swelling. Prednisone and dapsone were prescribed. The redness of the eyes resolved and marked improvement in the pain and swelling of the ears occurred.

Question: What is the diagnosis?

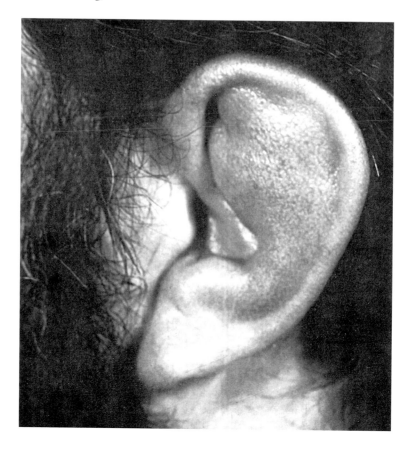

Diagnosis: Relapsing polychondritis with auricular chondritis and scleritis.

Discussion: Relapsing polychondritis is a rare inflammatory condition of unknown etiology affecting the cartilaginous portions of the ears, nose, trachea, and joints. The inflammatory process causes unilateral or bilateral acute painful swelling of the external ear that characteristically spares the ear lobule (see Figure), nasal septal cartilage loss resulting in a saddle-nose deformity, respiratory symptoms of hoarseness, wheezing, and dyspnea from inflammation of the tracheal cartilage, and a nonerosive, seronegative arthritis affecting small and large joints. Ocular complications of relapsing polychondritis include scleritis and episcleritis as in the present patient, and conjunctivitis, iridocyclitis, chorioretinitis, cataract, corneal infiltrates and corneal melting. The heart (aortic valve dysfunction) and kidneys (glomerulonephritis) are affected less commonly. Some patients have a systemic vasculitis, and nearly one-third have an associated autoimmune disorder, such as systemic lupus erythematosus, rheumatoid arthritis, Sjögren's syndrome, or spondyloarthropathy. Relapsing polychondritis may occur as a paraneoplastic syndrome associated with myelodysplastic disorders.

The differential diagnosis of chondritis includes infection (streptococcal, fungal, syphilitic, and lepromatous), trauma, neoplasm, and Wegener's granulomatosis. Biopsy of cartilage of patients with relapsing polychondritis shows a cellular infiltrate of mononuclear and polymorphonuclear cells and destructive changes in the fibrocartilage. Biopsy is not required in classic cases but serves to exclude other causes of chondritis when the diagnosis is problematic. Humoral and cellular immune responses to type II, type IX and type XI collagen have been described.

The present patient had bilateral auricular chondritis with scleritis and episcleritis. Stenosis of the external auditory canal resulted from auricular chondritis and caused mild hearing loss. He responded promptly to corticosteroid therapy, and dapsone was added for additional anti-inflammatory effect. Tracheal involvement, which this patient did not have, is one of the more serious complications of relapsing polychondritis and when present may require high-dose corticosteroids, immunosuppressive drugs, tracheotomy and stent placement if the trachea collapses.

Clinical Pearls

1. Relapsing polychondritis is a rare multisystem disease with chondritis as a prominent clinical feature.

2. Relapsing polychondritis may coexist with another autoimmune disease such as SLE, RA, and Sjögren's syndrome, or it may present as a paraneoplastic syndrome in association with myelodysplastic disorders.

3. An immune response against collagens II, IX, and XI has been demonstrated in many patients with relapsing polychondritis.

REFERENCES

1. Van Besien K, Tricot G, Hoffman R. Relapsing polychondritis: a paraneoplastic syndrome associated with myelodysplastic syndromes. Am J Hematol 1992;40:47–50.
2. Trentham DE. Relapsing polychondritis. In: McCarty DJ (ed): Arthritis and Allied Conditions. A Textbook of Rheumatology. Philadelphia, Lea & Febiger, 1993, pp 1369–1375.
3. Yang CL, Brinckmann J, Rui HF, et al. Autoantibodies to cartilage collagens in relapsing polychondritis. Arch Dermatol Res 1993;285:245–249.
4. Dunne JA, Sabanathan S. Use of metallic stents in relapsing polychondritis. Chest 1994;105:864–867.

PATIENT 4

A 16-year-old boy with weight loss, fever, and a dilated aorta

A 16-year-old boy presented with a 6-month history of anorexia, weight loss, and right arm pain with weakness. There was no significant past medical history. He had been sexually active and used marijuana daily, but denied IV drug use.

Physical Examination: Temperature 101°, other vital signs normal. Vascular: all pulses palpable and without bruits. Musculoskeletal: right arm tenderness with mild proximal muscle weakness.

Laboratory Findings: Hct 30%; WBC 12,400/μL with 68% PMNs, 21% neutrophils, and 11% monocytes; platelets 435,000/μL; ESR 66 mm/hr. Urinalysis: negative. Creatinine 0.7 mg/dL; ANA: neg; RF: 169 IU/mL (0–20); VDRL: negative; HIV Ab: negative; Hepatitis B and C antibodies: negative; CPK: 39 IU/mL. Chest radiograph: normal cardiac silhouette with a markedly tortuous thoracic aorta. Electromyogram: chronic myopathy of the right biceps muscle. Nerve conduction velocities: normal. Echocardiogram: normal. MRI of chest and abdomen: see Figure.

Question: What is the diagnosis?

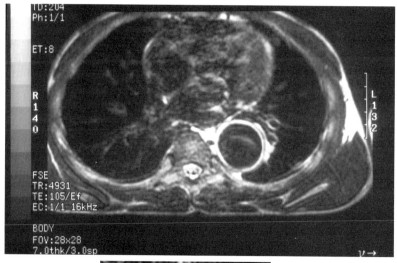

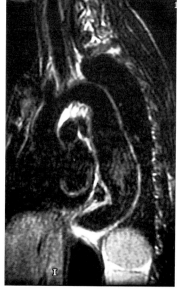

Diagnosis: Takayasu's artertis in the prepulseless stage.

Discussion: Takayasu's arteritis is a chronic, granulomatous inflammatory condition affecting the aorta and the proximal segments of its immediate branches. Although it is described most commonly in Japan, its distribution is worldwide. The ratio of females to males afflicted is approximately 4:1, most commonly patients are between 12 and 30 years of age. The etiology is unknown, but anti-aorta antibodies have been described in some patients.

The clinical course of Takayasu's arteritis is divided into two stages—prepulseless and pulseless. During the prepulseless stage, constitutional symptoms (fatigue, weight loss, and low-grade fever) are common and sometimes associated with a mild arthritis. During this stage, there may be a mild normochromic, normocytic anemia, elevated ESR, and polyclonal increase in gammaglobulins.

The pulseless stage is characterized by arterial vascular insufficiency due to large artery narrowing. At this time, the inflammatory period of the illness has resolved and the ESR is normal. Claudication, ischemic ulcers, Raynaud's phenomenon, and gangrene of extremities can occur. Bruits may be detected over the carotid and subclavian arteries, and pulses are diminished or absent. Hypertension may develop secondary to narrowing of the aorta or renal artery. In late stages of the illness, cerebral perfusion defects result in vertigo, syncope, strokes, seizures, and loss of vision. Abdominal angina or gastrointestinal bleeding may result from mesenteric artery involvement.

The aortic dilatation seen in the prepulseless stage of Takayasu's artertis must be differentiated from other causes of aortic aneurysm. Other illnesses are unlikely to involve the entire aorta as does Takayasu's arteritis. Ascending aortic involvement is seen in patients with syphilis, Marfan's syndrome, or seronegative spondyloarthropathies; more distal aneurysms may be a result of atherosclerotic diseases. The pulseless stage of Takayasu's artertis must be differentiated from arteritis of medium-sized vessels (polyarteritis nodosa), Buerger's disease, and severe atherosclerosis.

Establishing a diagnosis of prepulseless Takayasu's arteritis can be problematic as symptoms are nonspecific. An enlarged mediastinum on chest radiograph may be a clue. Aortography can reveal the dilated aorta, but MRI scanning is less invasive and confirms the diagnosis. The finding of panaortic dilatation or aortic wall thickening in a young person with systemic inflammatory symptoms and signs is considered to be diagnostic of Takayasu's artertis.

Treatment of prepulseless Takayasu's artertis involves the initial use of daily high-dose prednisone (1mg/kg/d) with subsequent tapering after several weeks, using symptoms and the ESR as guides. Long-term use of low-dose prednisone may help prevent long-term complications and the frequent relapses seen after discontinuation of corticosteroids. Occasionally, a cytotoxic drug must be added to the corticosteroids to control the inflammatory phase of the disease. In the pulseless stages of the disease, arterial bypass grafts or balloon dilatation may be needed to alleviate ischemic symptoms.

The present patient's constitutional symptoms and laboratory values were consistent with inflammation usually seen in prepulseless Takayasu's artertis. The diagnosis was confirmed by the MRI finding of dilatation throughout the aorta (see Figure). Therapy was initiated with prednisone, 1 mg/kg/d, and 2 months following its initiation his constitutional symptoms had resolved and the ESR was 16 mm/hr.

Clinical Pearls

1. The prepulseless stage of Takayasu's arteritis is characterized by nonspecific symptoms of inflammation and thickening and/or dilatation of the entire aorta.

2. MRI scanning of the chest and abdomen is most useful for the diagnosis of Takaysu's arteritis during the prepulseless stage.

3. Initial treatment of Takayasu's arteritis is oral corticosteroids (1mg prednisone/kg/d), using symptoms and the ESR to guide steroid tapering.

4. Takayasu's arteritis of long duration is characterized by symptoms of stenosis of the major aortic branches.

REFERENCES

1. Hall S, Barr W, Lie JT, et al. Takaysu's arteritis: a study of 32 North American patients. Medicine (Baltimore) 1985;64:89–99.
2. Yamato M, Lecky JW, Hiramatsu K, et al. Takaysu's arteritis: radiographic and angiographic findings in 59 patients. Radiology 1986;161:329–334.
3. Yamada I, Numano F, Suzuki S. Takayasu arteritis: evaluation with MR imaging. Radiology 1993;188:89–94.

PATIENT 5

A 45-year-old man with progressive weakness, hypoesthesias, lymphadenopathy, and gynecomastia

A 45-year-old man presented with weakness and hypoesthesia of the extremities. He was well until 4 months earlier when he developed diplopia and numbness of the face. A neurologic work-up was unrewarding, and he was diagnosed as having complex migraine headaches. He subsequently developed numbness and weakness beginning in the toes and gradually ascending to involve the legs and arms. He had lost 27 pounds but denied fever, chills, or night sweats. There was a past history of low back pain and two lumbar laminectomies. He denied drug or alcohol abuse.

Physical Examination: Temperature 97.8°; pulse 86; respirations 20; blood pressure 150/80. Skin: normal. Lymph nodes: enlarged, nontender cervical and inguinal nodes. HEENT: normal. Chest: bilateral gynecomastia. Lungs: normal. Cardiovascular: normal. Abdomen: nontender. Rectal: normal sphincter tone with guaiac negative stool. Musculoskeletal: full ROM of all joints and no synovitis. Neurologic: alert and oriented; cranial nerves II-XII intact; gait ataxic; finger-to-nose test normal; distal weakness and decreased motor tone affecting legs more than arms; absent DTRs; absent sensation to light touch below knees, and diminished pinprick and vibratory sensation in lower extremities.

Laboratory Findings: Hct 44%; WBC 6,600/μL with 64% neutrophils, 10% lymphocytes, 14% atypical lymphocytes, 9% monocytes, 1% eosinophils, 2% basophils; platelets 920,000/μL; ESR 65 mm/hr. Electrolytes: normal; glucose 129 mg/dL; TFT's normal; CPK normal; serum protein electrophoresis (see Figure). Urinalysis: microscopic negative, total protein 294 mg/24 hrs, Bence-Jones protein negative, electrophoresis normal, heavy metal screen negative. B12 and folate normal; ANA negative; ANCA negative; HBSag negative; HIV negative. CSF: no cells, glucose 77 mg/dL, protein 333 mg/dL, VDRL negative, cultures and stains negative. Chest radiograph: normal. ECG and echocardiogram: normal. Renal biopsy: normal. CT scan of chest and abdomen: bilateral gynecomastia and pleural effusions, multiple mediastinal and abdominal lymph nodes. Bone survey: no lytic or sclerotic lesions. Electromyelogram and nerve conduction velocity study: mixed axonal and demyelinating neuropathy of all four extremities. Bone marrow examination: multiple nodules of plasma cells that stained positive for lambda light chains and negative for kappa light chains. Sural nerve biopsy: axonal degeneration and segmental demyelination; non-necrotizing epineurial vasculitis; epineurial and endoneurial deposits with apple-green birefringence under polarizing microscopy.

Question: What is the diagnosis?

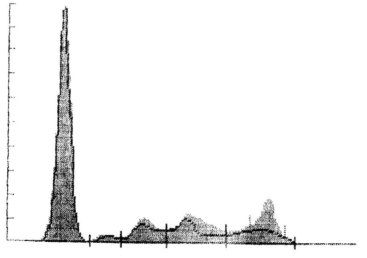

005

Diagnosis: Plasma cell dyscrasia with polyneuropathy or incomplete POEMS syndrome.

Discussion: Peripheral neuropathy is associated with a plasma-cell dyscrasia in up to 10% of cases. Plasma-cell dyscrasias with polyneuropathy include nonmalignant monoclonal gammopathies, multiple myeloma, Waldenström's macroglobulinemia, amyloidosis, osteosclerotic myeloma, and the POEMS syndrome. **POEMS** syndrome is defined as **P**olyneuropathy, **O**rganomegaly (splenomegaly, hepatomegaly, or lymphadenopathy), **E**ndocrinopathy (hypogonadism, hypothyroidism, or diabetes mellitus), **M**onoclonal gammopathy, and **S**kin changes (hyperpigmentation, hypertrichosis, scleroderma-like thickening, peripheral edema). POEMS syndrome occurs in men more frequently than in women, with an average age of onset of 46 years. Sclerotic bone lesions are often present in POEMS syndrome, and there is significant clinical and histopathologic overlap with *osteosclerotic* myeloma. Unlike multiple myeloma, the bone lesions seen in polyneuropathy with plasma-cell dyscrasia are sclerotic, not lytic, and usually painless.

The polyneuropathy accompanying plasma-cell dyscrasia is predominantly demyelinating and typically presents as a distal, symmetric sensorimotor deficit with progressive proximal involvement. Motor and sensory nerve conduction velocities are slowed, and nerve biopsy reveals degeneration of myelin sheaths and axons. Cerebrospinal fluid protein levels are nearly always elevated, often more than 200 mg/dL and usually with a normal cell count.

An M component (IgG or IgA) is present in the serum of up to 90% of patients with POEMS syndrome but is usually not detected in urine. Unlike multiple myeloma where kappa light chains outnumber lambda light chains by 2:1, in POEMS syndrome or polyneuropathy with plasma-cell dyscrasia the M component nearly always contains lambda light chains.

The present patient had **P**olyneuropathy, **O**rganomegaly (lymphadenopathy), **E**ndocrinopathy (gynecomastia and diabetes), **M** protein (see Figure), but did **not** have **S**kin changes at presentation—thus, the diagnosis of incomplete POEMS syndrome or polyneuropathy with plasma-cell dyscrasia. As shown in the Figure, there is a small M spike present in the gamma fraction of the serum protein electrophoresis measuring 0.99 g/dL. Immunoelectrophoresis identified the M spike as IgG lambda. In contrast to multiple myeloma, the patient had lymphadenopathy and endocrinopathy and did not have painful lytic bone lesions. Although amyloid deposition was seen in the sural nerve biopsy specimen, this patient was younger and did not have features of primary amyloidosis, i.e., macroglossia, cardiomyopathy, nephrosis, or autonomic dysfunction.

Patients with incomplete POEMS syndrome appear to have the same clinical outcome as those with the complete form. Like osteosclerotic myeloma, the course is often indolent and the five-year survival rate is 60%, compared to 20% for patients with multiple myeloma. Treatment options include local radiation, alkylating agents, corticosteroids and plasmapheresis, but death often results from progressive polyneuropathy and complications such as pneumonia or sepsis.

The present patient was treated with melphalan and prednisone and experienced slow progression of the polyneuropathy.

Clinical Pearls

1. Peripheral neuropathy occurs in nearly 10% of plasma-cell dyscrasias and may be the presenting manifestation.

2. POEMS syndrome is a rare condition in which a plasma-cell dyscrasia occurs in association with **P**olyneuropathy, **O**rganomegaly, **E**ndocrinopathy, **M**onoclonal gammopathy, and **S**kin changes.

3. Unlike multiple myeloma, bone lesions, if present, are usually asymptomatic and sclerotic, not painful and lytic.

4. Some patients have an incomplete form of POEMS syndrome that has considerable overlap with osteosclerotic myeloma.

5. The M protein nearly always contains lambda light chains in patients with POEMS syndrome.

REFERENCES

1. Bardwick PA, Zvaifler NJ, Gill GN, et al. Plasma cell dyscrasia with polyneuropathy, organomegaly, endocrinopathy, M protein, and skin changes: the POEMS syndrome: report on two cases and a review of the literature. Medicine (Baltimore) 1980; 59:311–322.
2. Case Records of the Massachusetts General Hospital (Case 39–1992). N Engl J Med 1992;327:1014–1021.
3. Miralles, GD, O'Fallon JR, Talley NJ. Plasma-cell dyscrasia with polyneuropathy. The spectrum of the POEMS syndrome. N Engl J Med 1992;327:1919–1923.

PATIENT 6

A 37-year-old woman with arthritis and a history of thrombocytopenia

A 37-year-old woman reported painful swelling of the MCP, PIP, and MTP joints of 3 months' duration. She had morning stiffness lasting 2 hours, fatigue, and low-grade late afternoon fever, but denied oral ulcers, alopecia, and photosensitivity. Two years earlier she was treated with prednisone and splenectomy for thrombocytopenia.

Physical Examination: Joints: swelling and tenderness of the PIP and MCP joints of both hands; tenderness of the MTP joints of both feet.

Laboratory Findings: Hct 42%; WBC 8,100/μL with 60% neutrophils, 28% lymphocytes, 5% monocytes, 5% eosinophils, 2% basophils; platelets 376,000/μL; PT 12.3 sec; PTT 31.2 sec. Urinalysis: trace protein, no erythrocytes or leukocytes. Creatinine: 0.7 mg/dL. ANA: positive at 1:640 (speckled pattern). Anti-double stranded DNA: positive at 1:10. Anti-Smith antibody: negative. VDRL: positive at 1:2. MHATP (treponemal-specific test): negative. Lupus anticoagulant: negative. Anti-cardiolipin antibodies: IgG negative, IgM positive at 15.

Question: What is the diagnosis?

Diagnosis: Systemic lupus erythematosus with antiphospholipid antibody syndrome.

Discussion: Systemic lupus erythematosus (SLE), an autoimmune disease with manifestations in many organ systems, most often presents with arthritis, rash, pleuritis, or renal involvement. However, the initial manifestation may be hematologic, such as lymphopenia, neutropenia, thrombocytopenia, or anemia. Initially, patients may have no other symptoms, signs, or laboratory abnormalities to suggest SLE other than immune mediated thrombocytopenia or hemolysis. These patients are diagnosed as idiopathic thrombocytopenia (ITP) or Evan's syndrome and treated accordingly. Over time the patient accrues additional manifestations that make the underlying connective tissue disease apparent.

Thrombocytopenia in SLE can result from several causes. Classically, it is immune-mediated, with circulating anti-platelet antibodies, and usually responds to high-dose corticosteroids. However, treatment with intravenous gamma globulin or immunosuppression with cytotoxic agents may be required in some patients. Thrombotic thrombocytopenia purpura (TTP), which may be seen in SLE, is characterized by thrombocytopenia, microangiopathic hemolytic anemia (with schistocytes evident on peripheral smear), renal disease, fever, and mental status changes. Treatment of TTP usually requires plasmapheresis.

Certain drugs used to treat SLE, such as azathioprine or cyclophosphamide, may result in thrombocytopenia due to bone marrow supression. In such cases, the thrombocytopenia is usually accompanied by neutropenia, and withdrawal of the medication with reinstitution at a lower dose is often adequate to control the thrombocytopenia.

There is an association of immune thrombocytopenia with the presence of the antiphospholipid or lupus anticoagulant syndrome. In this syndrome, recurrent venous or arterial thromboses, recurrent fetal loss, or thrombocytopenia are seen. A number of tests may indicate the presence of antibodies to phospholipids. Because the older serologic tests for syphilis, such as the VDRL, are dependent on detecting antibodies to phospholipid, they are often positive in the face of a negative treponemal specific test in this condition (false-positive serologic test for syphilis). The term "anticoagulant" comes from the fact that there is often prolongation of the partial thromboplastin time (PTT), which is not corrected by mixing with normal plasma, indicating the presence of an inhibitor rather than a factor deficiency. It is important to recognize that this is not an actual anticoagulant, as these patients are predisposed to thrombosis. The anticardiolipin test uses an ELISA test to detect antibodies (either IgG or IgM) to this phospholipid. The results of the lupus anticoagulant test and the antiphospholipid test differ often enough that both tests should be performed when this condition is suspected.

Treatment of the antiphospholipid syndrome is controversial, but most authorities now agree that prolonged anticoagulation is justified in those patients who have had recurrent episodes of thrombosis. Treatment with antiplatelet doses of aspirin or treatment with subcutaneous heparin have been used in pregnant women with antiphospholipid antibodies and a history of recurrent fetal loss.

In the present patient, the development of arthritis and the findings of antinuclear and anti-DNA antibodies established the diagnosis of systemic lupus erythematosus, which was not evident at the time of her thrombocytopenia and splenectomy. She was treated with a nonsteroidal anti-inflammatory agent for arthritis and a baby aspirin daily.

Clinical Pearls

1. Thrombocytopenia may be the presenting manifestation of systemic lupus erythematosus, with other features of the disease becoming evident later.

2. Thrombocytopenia in SLE may be associated with the presence of circulating antibodies to phospholipid, which are detected by tests for the lupus anticoagulant and anticardiolipin antibody.

3. Treatment of the antiphospholipid antibody syndrome includes prolonged anticoagulation for those patients with recurrent episodes of thrombosis, and antiplatelet agents and/or heparin for women with a history of recurrent fetal loss.

REFERENCES

1. Harris EN. Thrombosis, recurrent fetal loss, and thrombocytopenia: Predictive value of the anticardiolipin antibody test. Arch Intern Med 1986;146:2153–2156.
2. Lockshin MD, Qamar T, Druzin ML, et al. Antibody to cardiolipin, lupus anticoagulant and fetal death. J Rheumatol 1987;14:259–262.
3. Alarcon-Segovia D, Deleze M, Oria CV. Antiphospholipid antibodies and the antiphospholipid syndrome in systemic lupus erythematosus. A prospective analysis of 500 consecutive patients. Medicine (Baltimore) 1989;68:353–365.

PATIENT 7

A 78-year-old woman with knee and ankle pain following parathyroidectomy

A 78-year-old woman was admitted for resection of a parathyroid adenoma. While undergoing evaluation for a 25-pound weight loss, she had been found to have hypercalcemia (10.9 mg/dL) and hypophosphatemia (2.6 mg/dL), with normal renal function. A serum parathyroid hormone level was elevated.

Physical Examination: Normal.

Laboratory Findings: Normal.

Hospital Course: Two days after resection of a right superior parathyroid adenoma, the patient complained of right knee and ankle pain. Both joints were warm and swollen with decreased range of motion. Radiographs of the foot showed osteopenia with osteophyte formation, and a radiograph of the knee is shown below. Arthrocentesis of the knee yielded a small amount of cloudy synovial fluid that demonstrated crystals with weakly positive birefringence when examined under compensated polarizing light microscopy. Her serum calcium was 8.2 mg/dL, serum urate was normal, and urinalysis was unrevealing.

Question: What are the radiographic findings in the knee and what is the diagnosis?

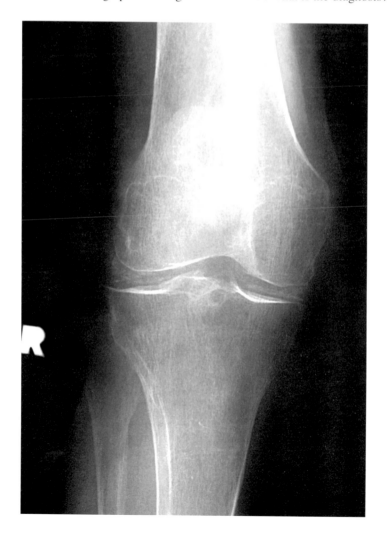

Diagnosis: Chondrocalcinosis with postparathyroidectomy pseudogout.

Discussion: Chondrocalcinosis refers to the deposition of calcium pyrophosphate dihydrate (CPPD) within hyaline cartilage and fibrocartilage. Chondrocalcinosis may be an asymptomatic radiographic finding or may be associated with acute crystal-induced synovitis (pseudogout) or chronic arthropathy. The prevalence of chondrocalcinosis increases with age, and nearly 33% of those over 75 years of age have radiographic chondrocalcinosis of the knees. A number of metabolic and endocrine abnormalities have been associated with chondrocalcinosis. Taking into account age as a confounding variable, the following conditions are associated with an increased prevalence of chondrocalcinosis: hyperparathyroidism, hemochromatosis, hypophosphatasia, hypomagnesemia, and possibly hypothyroidism. Pseudogout may occur in any of these conditions or in the normal elderly patient. Hemochromatosis is associated not only with chondrocalcinosis and pseudogout but also with a chronic destructive arthropathy. There is less convincing evidence to support an association between chondrocalcinosis and gout, diabetes mellitus, Wilson's disease, and ochronosis.

CPPD crystal formation is promoted by elevation of either calcium or inorganic pyrophosphate. Synovial fluid levels of pyrophosphate are elevated in patients with hyperparathyroidism, hemochromatosis, and hypomagnesemia. In addition to elevated levels of pyrophosphate, the hypercalcemia present in hyperparathyroidism serves to promote CPPD crystal formation and deposition in cartilage. Calcium moves easily into and out of cartilage and in the event of hypocalcemia, CPPD crystals may become soluble and be shed into the synovial space, where an acute inflammatory synovitis (pseudogout) ensues.

Chondrocalcinosis exists as punctate or linear densities in articular hyaline or fibrocartilage. Within the knee, chondrocalcinosis is characteristically present in the articular cartilage, meniscus, or articular capsule. The radiograph of the present patient reveals chondrocalcinosis within the articular cartilage and meniscus (see Figure). Other common radiographic sites of chondrocalcinosis include the articular fibrocartilage of the wrist, the symphysis pubis, the acetabular labrum of the hip joint, and the anulus fibrosus of the intervertebral discs.

Serum calcium, phosphorus, alkaline phosphatase, magnesium, and possibly thyroid function tests should be obtained in any patient with chondrocalcinosis. In men younger than 55 years, hemochromatosis should be excluded. Asymptomatic chondrocalcinosis requires no treatment. Attacks of pseudogout, as in the present patient, can be managed with nonsteroidal anti-inflammatory drugs or injection of affected joints with corticosteroids. Treatment of any associated metabolic condition does not alter the course of CPPD deposition disease.

The present patient was treated with a nonsteroidal anti-inflammatory agent and the joint symptoms resolved. The serum calcium returned to normal.

Clinical Pearls

1. Chondrocalcinosis is the result of calcium pyrophosphate dihydrate (CPPD) crystal deposition within hyaline cartilage or fibrocartilage.

2. A dramatic increase in the prevalence of chondrocalcinosis occurs with increasing age, and over 30% of persons over 75 years have chondrocalcinosis of the knees.

3. Chondrocalcinosis and pseudogout are associated with hyperparathyroidism, hemochromatosis, hypomagnesemia, hypophosphatasia, and possibly hypothyroidism.

4. Radiographic screening for chondrocalcinosis can be accomplished with a single anteroposterior (AP) view of both knees, an AP view of the pelvis for hips and symphysis pubis, and a single posteroanterior view of both hands and wrists.

5. Postparathyroidectomy pseudogout is likely the result of hypocalcemia and solubilization of cartilaginous CPPD crystals that are then shed into the joint space.

REFERENCES

1. Bilezikian JP, Aurbach GD, Connor TB. Pseudogout after parathyroidectomy. Lancet 1973;1:445–446.
2. Doherty M, Chuck A, Hosking D, et al. Inorganic pyrophosphate in metabolic diseases predisposing to calcium pyrophosphate dihydrate crystal deposition. Arthritis Rheum 1991;34:1297–1303.
3. Jones AC, Chuck AJ, Arie EA, et al. Diseases associated with calcium pyrophosphate deposition disease. Sem Arthritis Rheum 1992;22:188–202.

PATIENT 8

A 61-year-old woman with rheumatoid arthritis and chest pain

A 61-year-old woman with rheumatoid arthritis for 3 years on methotrexate (15 mg per week), naproxen (500 mg bid), and prednisone (5 mg per day) developed chest pain 3 days before presentation. She initially noted 1 hour of chest discomfort and a sore throat. The pain was not caused by exertion and subsided over 1 hour. One day later she noted anterior chest pain with radiation into the neck, nausea, and diaphoresis. The pain was improved on sitting up, but was not related to exertion or eating.

Physical Examination: Blood pressure 100/76 with pulsus paradoxus 8 mmHg; heart rate 110, respiratory rate 16. Cardiovascular: normal heart sounds without pericardial rub.

Laboratory Findings: WBC 21,800/µL; Hct 31%. Creatine kinase: normal on three occasions. Chest radiograph: normal. ECG (shown below).

Question: What is the cause of the patient's chest pain?

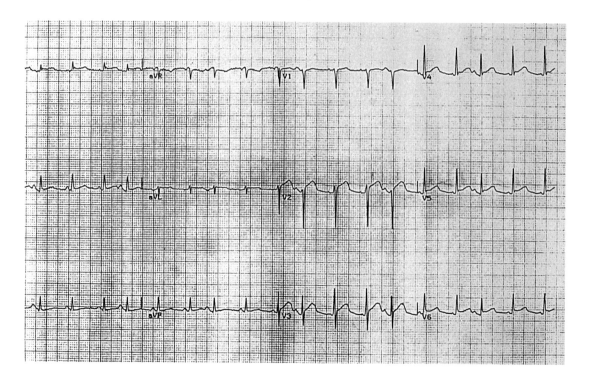

Diagnosis: Rheumatoid pericarditis.

Discussion: Although histopathologic evidence of pericarditis is extremely common in autopsies of patients with rheumatoid arthritis, clinical pericarditis occurs in a minority of patients. With the advent of echocardiography, it has become clear that many patients with rheumatoid arthritis have small- to medium-sized pericardial effusions that are asymptomatic. Women are affected more often than men, and the occurrence is positively correlated with the titer of the rheumatoid factor. When symptoms are present, pericardial inflammation is manifested as chest pain, heart failure, or a pericardial friction rub. When evaluated chemically, the pericardial fluid is characterized by low or absent glucose and elevated protein levels. Rheumatoid pericarditis may be complicated by tamponade or chronic constrictive pericarditis.

The presence of rheumatoid arthritis does not alter the general clinical approach to the evaluation of chest pain. Coronary insufficiency in rheumatoid arthritis patients is usually a result of atherosclerosis, which occurs at an increased frequency in this population. Coronary insufficiency from rheumatoid vasculitis rarely occurs and should be considered in only unusual instances because of the different therapeutic implications of this diagnosis. Valvular rheumatoid disease is also exceedingly rare, although rheumatoid nodules can result in aortic incompetence and conduction defects.

Treatment of symptomatic rheumatoid pericarditis includes high-dose oral corticosteroids (prednisone at 1 mg/kg/d). Symptoms usually subside over a few days followed by echocardiographic resolution of pericardial fluid over several weeks. In some patients, pericardiectomy is needed to relieve constrictive pericarditis.

The present patient was treated with 60 mg of prednisone daily with resolution of symptoms in several days. A follow-up echocardiogram at 1 month showed that the pericardial effusion had resolved.

Clinical Pearls

1. Although a frequent autopsy or echocardiographic finding, rheumatoid pericarditis is not commonly symptomatic.

2. Coronary artery insufficiency in patients with rheumatoid arthritis is usually due to atherosclerotic disease rather than to coronary arteritis, which is rare.

3. When pericardial fluid is aspirated from a rheumatoid effusion, the glucose level is low as seen in rheumatoid pleurisy.

4. Patients with rheumatoid pericarditis have a rapid clinical response to high dose oral corticosteroids.

5. Pericardiectomy is sometimes required for constrictive pericarditis.

REFERENCES
1. Lebowitz WB. The heart in RA (Rheumatoid disease): A clinical and pathological study of 62 cases. Ann Intern Med 1963;58:102–106.
2. Thadani U, Iveson JMI, Wright V. Cardiac tamponade, constrictive pericarditis, and pericardial resection in RA. Medicine 1975;54:261–270.
3. Hara KS, Ballard DJ, Ilstrum DM, et al. Rheumatoid pericarditis: Clinical features and survival. Medicine 1990;69:81–91.

PATIENT 9

A 3-year-old girl with arthritis, uveitis, and skin lesions

A 3-year-old girl developed painless swelling of the wrists and ankles unresponsive to salicylates. She was referred for rheumatologic evaluation at the age of 4, when bilateral granulomatous uveitis and posterior synechiae were noted. Glaucoma developed in the right eye despite treatment with ophthalmic and oral corticosteroids, and visual acuity did not improve with iridectomy.

Physical Examination: Vital signs: normal. Skin: hypopigmented 2- to 3-mm papules on the thighs. Lymph nodes: normal. HEENT: irregular pupils with decreased visual acuity. Extremities: both wrists and ankles swollen with full range of motion.

Laboratory Findings: CBC normal; serum chemistries normal; RF and ANA negative. Radiographs of the wrists and ankles: soft tissue swelling without bony abnormalities. Chest radiograph: normal. Serum angiotensin-converting enzyme (ACE) level: normal. A skin biopsy was performed (Figure).

Question: What is the diagnosis?

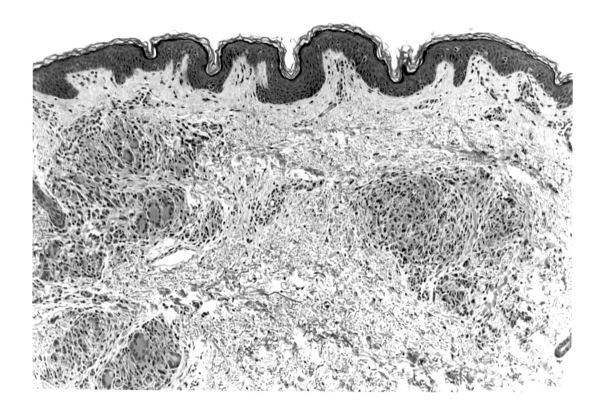

Diagnosis: Childhood-onset sarcoidosis.

Discussion: Sarcoidosis is a chronic, multisystem, granulomatous disorder of unknown cause that occurs most commonly between 20 and 40 years of age. Childhood sarcoidosis is rare and has two subsets of patients. Children between ages 8 and 15 years virtually always have lung disease and may have eye, skin, liver, and spleen involvement. Children younger than 6 years (preschool sarcoidosis) have a classic triad of arthritis, uveitis, and skin rash *without* pulmonary involvement or elevated ACE levels.

Arthritis, as in the present patient, may be the presenting manifestation in young children. A diagnosis of pauci-articular juvenile arthritis (JRA) is often made, since this juvenile arthritis subtype typically affects young children and may be complicated by uveitis. Joint involvement of childhood sarcoidosis differs from that of JRA in several aspects. In childhood sarcoidosis, most of the joint swelling appears to be due to extensor tenosynovitis rather than arthritis; despite swelling, range of motion is well-preserved. The degree of pain experienced by children with sarcoidosis is less than that of children with JRA. Radiographic changes are minimal in sarcoidosis compared with the extensive cartilage loss and bony erosion that may occur in JRA.

Ocular involvement occurs in over 60% of children with sarcoidosis, at an average age of onset of 3 years, yet sarcoidosis is an uncommon cause of uveitis in children. JRA is the most common systemic illness associated with anterior uveitis in children, accounting for more than 80% of cases in some series. In JRA, uveitis is characteristically nongranulomatous, rarely involves the posterior segment, and usually is associated with antinuclear antibodies (ANA). The uveitis of childhood sarcoidosis may be granulomatous or nongranulomatous, may involve the posterior segment, and is almost never associated with ANA.

Joint and ocular features of childhood sarcoidosis mimic those of JRA, but the skin lesions are distinctive. The skin manifestations of sarcoidosis are protean but should never be confused with the typical exanthem of JRA (evanescent salmon-colored macules and urticarial papules). Moreover, the rash of JRA is seen in children with the systemic-onset type (Still's disease), not in the subset of children with pauci-articular onset who are at greatest risk for uveitis. In childhood sarcoidosis, the skin examination may show confluent papules, eczematous or ichthyosiform dermatitis, exfoliative erythroderma, dermal and subcutaneous nodules, and symmetric maculopapular eruptions. The present patient exhibited confluent papules, and a skin biopsy specimen (see Figure) revealed intradermal granulomas composed predominantly of epithelioid histiocytes and a small number of lymphocytes and foreign body-type giant cells. Special stains for acid-fast bacilli and fungi were negative.

The present patient's tenosynovitis was unresponsive to salicylates, nonsteroidal anti-inflammatory drugs and corticosteroid injections. Her uveitis was treated with oral and topical steroids and cycloplegics, but was complicated by secondary glaucoma and cataracts.

Clinical Pearls

1. Unlike sarcoidosis in adults and older children, early-onset (<6 years) childhood sarcoidosis is characterized by the triad of joint, eye and skin disease usually *without* pulmonary involvement or elevated ACE levels.

2. Features that distinguish early-onset sarcoidosis from JRA include boggy synovitis with little pain and preserved joint range of motion, granulomatous and posterior uveitis, absence of ANA, and distinctive skin lesions containing granulomas.

3. The outcome of early-onset sarcoidosis is dictated by the eye disease more than the joint or skin disease.

REFERENCES

1. Hetherington S. Sarcoidosis in young children. Am J Dis Child 1982;136:13–15.
2. Hoover DL, Khan JA, Giangiacomo J. Pediatric ocular sarcoidosis. Surv Ophthalmol 1986;30:215–228.
3. Sahn EE, Hampton MT, Garen PD, et al. Preschool sarcoidosis masquerading as juvenile rheumatoid arthritis: two case reports and a review of the literature. Pediatr Dermatol 1990;7:208–213.
4. Mathur A, Kremer JM. Immunopathology, rheumatic features, and therapy of sarcoidosis. Curr Opin Rheumatol 1992;4:76–80.

PATIENT 10

A 66-year-old man with testicular swelling

A 66-year-old man with a history of coronary artery disease and hypertension developed fatigue and low-grade fevers of 101° to 103°. He had a 2-month history of intermittent, painful testicular swelling that did not respond to tetracycline therapy for epididymitis. Subsequently, he developed night sweats and weight loss.

Physical Examination: Temperature: 101°. General appearance: chronically ill. Skin: tender subcutaneous nodules on the extremities with overlying erythema. Genitalia: scrotum erythematous with swollen, tender testes.

Laboratory Findings: WBC 9,600/μL, Hct 32%, ESR 140 mm/hr. BUN 13 mg/dL; Creatinine 0.9 mg/dL. Liver function tests: normal. Albumin: 2.1 gm/dL. Complement components 3 and 4: normal. Antinuclear antibodies: negative. Antineutrophil cytoplasmic antibodies: negative. RPR: negative. HIV antibodies: negative. Hepatitis A, B, and C serology: negative. Blood cultures (6 sets): negative. Bone marrow biopsy: 16% plasma cells, otherwise normal. Serum protein electrophoresis: polyclonal hypergammaglobulinemia. Electromyography and nerve conduction studies: absent sural nerve conduction. Sural nerve biopsy: normal. Angiography of renal, hepatic and mesenteric arteries: normal. Skin biopsy: shown below.

Question: What is the diagnosis?

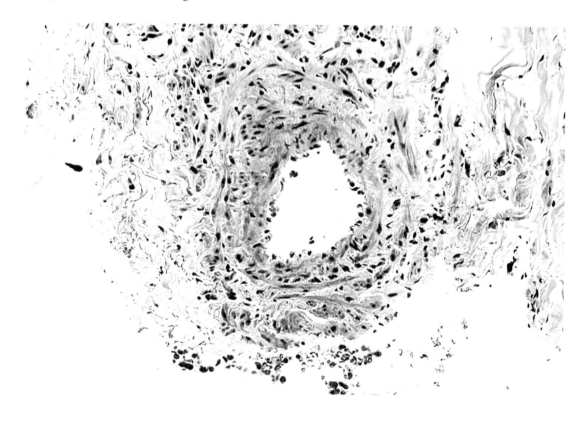

Diagnosis: Polyarteritis nodosa (PAN).

Discussion: Polyarteritis nodosa is an unusual disorder, occurring in less than 2 of 100,000 persons each year. It affects males more commonly than females by 2:1, and most frequently occurs during middle age. Characterized by a necrosing inflammation of all mural layers of medium-sized muscular arteries, the cause of PAN is unknown in the majority of patients. The pathophysiology, however, involves deposition of immune complexes in vessel walls and activation of humoral and cellular mediators of inflammation. In some cases, the antigen in these immune complexes is known to be hepatitis B. In regions where hepatitis B is endemic, the prevalence of polyarteritis nodosa is much increased. Polyarteritis also may be a complicating feature of collagen vascular disorders, such as rheumatoid arthritis, systemic lupus erythematosus, and Sjögren's syndrome, in addition to hairy cell leukemia.

The joints, kidneys, peripheral nerves and gastrointestinal tract can be affected to varying degrees. Patients may present with protean clinical manifestations, depending on which organs are most severely involved. There are usually constitutional features of fatigue, malaise, and weight loss. Dermal lesions include palpable purpura, livedo reticularis, ulcerations, and digital ischemia. Palpable subcutaneous nodules of up to several centimeters may be found along the extremities. The arthritis is an asymmetric, nondeforming polyarthritis of the lower extremity and is more common early in the disease course. Peripheral neuropathy occurs in up to 70% of patients and may be the presenting feature. The onset may be sudden and result in a foot or wrist drop characteristic of mononeuritis multiplex.

Renal involvement features hypertension and nephritis with microscopic hematuria and red blood cell casts. Progressive azotemia as a result of glomerulonephritis is common. Abdominal pain resulting from ischemia of a specific organ is the most common gastrointestinal symptom, and gastrointestinal bleeding may also result. Infarction of either the gallbladder or the appendix has been reported. Testicular involvement is manifested as pain, swelling, or induration and may be the presenting feature of the disease.

Laboratory tests are nonspecific but reflect the inflammation present. A normocytic anemia, hypoalbuminemia, elevated ESR, and thrombocytosis indicate activation of the acute phase response. There may be evidence of complement consumption with low $C3$ and $C4$ components. Hepatitis B surface antigenemia may exist in patients with PAN secondary to infection with this agent.

The diagnosis of polyarteritis nodosa usually depends on a histologic examination of tissue biopsied from an affected organ. Samples biopsied from a palpable nodule along an extremity usually show the characteristic fibrinoid necrosis of the arterial wall and perivascular inflammation. When involvement of the sural nerve is documented by electromyographic studies, nerve biopsy may demonstrate vasculitis in the vasa nervorum. Because there may be involvement of arteries in skeletal muscle, a simultaneous biopsy of the gastrocnemius muscle should be performed. Larger dermal vessels can be sampled with excisional biopsies. Testicular biopsy may show the vasculitis in clinically affected testes. Kidney biopsy is usually unable to obtain arteries of the size involved, revealing only focal segmental necrotizing glomerulonephritis. There is also the possibility that a percutaneous renal biopsy will hit a pseudoaneurysm and result in significant hemorrhage. For these reasons renal biopsy should be avoided.

In the absence of histologic evidence of vasculitis, arteriography of visceral vessels can be used to confirm the diagnosis of PAN. Renal, hepatic, and mesenteric arteries should be studied for saccular aneurysms and tapering of arteries.

The prognosis of untreated PAN is rather dismal, with 5-year survival rates of less than 15%. Thus aggressive treatment with high-dose oral corticosteroids and the alkylating agent cyclophosphamide is warranted. Cyclophosphamide should be administered as oral tablets on a daily basis, because intermittent intravenous administration is associated with a higher relapse rate. Treatment is usually continued for 1 year after resolution of active disease.

The present patient demonstrated a medium-sized muscular artery with mural necrosis and a perivascular infiltrate consisting of polymorphonuclear leukocytes on the skin biopsy sample confirming the diagnosis of PAN. He was treated with prednisone, 60 mg/day, and cyclophosphamide, 100 mg/day, with resolution of the constitutional symptoms and testicular swelling.

Clinical Pearls

1. Polyarteritis nodosa is a vasculitis involving medium-sized muscular arteries in multiple organs. The organs most commonly affected are the skin, kidneys, gastrointestinal tract, joints, and liver.

2. Hepatitis B infection is the most common known etiology for PAN, but it accounts for only a minority of cases except in high hepatitis prevalence areas or at risk populations, such as intravenous drug users.

3. Diagnosis of PAN is best made histologically by biopsy of an affected organ, such as a peripheral nerve, muscle, skin, or a palpable nodule. Alternatively, a diagnosis may be made by visceral angiography of renal, hepatic, and mesenteric arteries showing saccular aneurysms or tapering.

REFERENCES

1. Fauci AS, Katz P, Haynes BF, et al. Cyclophosphamide therapy of severe systemic necrotizing vasculitis. N Engl J Med. 1979;301:235–238.
2. Albert DA, Rimon D, Silverstein MC. The diagnosis of polyarterits nodosa. I: A literature-based decision analysis approach. Arthrits Rheum 1988; 31:1117–1127.
3. Hall S, Conn DL. Immunosuppressive therapy for vasculitis. Curr Opin Rheumatol 1995;7:25–29.

PATIENT 11

A 32-year-old woman with fever, arthritis, and rash

A 32-year-old woman presented with a 3-day history of low-grade fever followed by acute polyarthritis. Pain and swelling began in the knees and then involved the ankles, wrists, and hands. Several days later a rash was noted on her legs. The rash was described as painful, red "bumps" that were warm and very tender to touch. The patient had a history of rheumatic fever at age 19 without cardiac sequelae. Two weeks earlier her teeth were cleaned, at which time she received prophylactic penicillin. Oral contraceptive pills had been discontinued 1 month earlier.

Physical Examination: Temperature 100.6°; pulse 100 and regular; respirations 18; blood pressure 100/80. Skin: multiple warm and tender subcutaneous nodules on extensor surface of the lower legs; several nodules appeared ecchymotic. Nodes: normal. HEENT: normal. Chest: normal. Cardiac: normal. Abdomen: normal. Musculoskeletal: swollen, tender ankle joints with pain on flexion and extension; warmth and tenderness of the knees with moderate-sized effusions; mild synovitis of both wrists. Extremities: 1+ pitting pretibial edema.

Laboratory Findings: Hct 43%; WBC 9,700/μL with 66% neutrophils, 20% lymphocytes, 8% monocytes, 5% eosinophils, 1% basophils; platelet count 383,000/μL; ESR 65 mm/hr; C-reactive protein 12.1 mg/dL. ASO titer: 100 IU. Electrolytes and liver panel: normal. Amylase and lipase: normal. Urinalysis: normal. RF and ANA: negative. PPD skin test: negative. ECG: normal. Chest radiograph: see Figure. Ankle radiographs: soft tissue swelling without erosive changes.

Question: What are the diagnosis and prognosis for this patient?

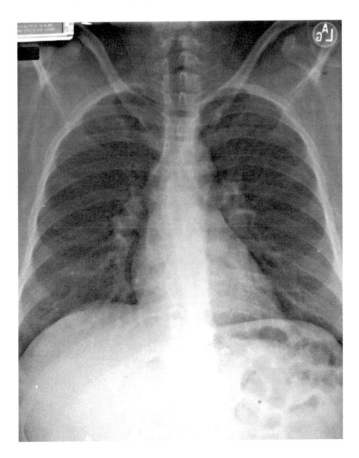

Diagnosis: Löfgren's syndrome with complete recovery.

Discussion: The triad of polyarthritis, erythema nodosum, and bilateral hilar adenopathy is known as Löfgren's syndrome. Nearly half of such patients have acute sarcoidosis. Other patients with erythema nodosum, sometimes in association with polyarthritis and hilar adenopathy, have an infectious process that is bacterial (streptococcal, tuberculosis, yersinia, leprosy, leptospirosis, tularemia, cat-scratch fever), fungal (coccidioidomycosis, blastomycosis, histoplasmosis), or viral (paravaccinia, infectious mononucleosis). Other associations with erythema nodosum, but not necessarily Löfgren's syndrome, include medications (sulfonamides, estrogen, oral contraceptives), inflammatory bowel disease, malignancy (lymphoma and leukemia), Behçet's syndrome, and pregnancy.

The prevalence of erythema nodosum varies widely among patients with acute sarcoid arthritis. The highest prevalence occurs in Scandinavia, where two-thirds of patients with acute or subacute sarcoid arthritis have associated erythema nodosum. Differences in prevalence of Löfgren's syndrome among patients with acute sarcoidosis may relate to immunogenetic factors. The HLA-B8,-DR3 haplotype may identify a group of patients who are more likely to have acute sarcoidosis and hilar adenopathy without developing chronic disease. Most patients with acute sarcoidosis presenting as Löfgren's syndrome have a self-limited course.

Acute sarcoid arthritis is a symmetric polyarthritis involving the ankles, knees, wrists, and small joints of the hands in decreasing frequency. Swelling of the ankles is more often due to tenosynovitis and periarticular soft tissue edema than to frank arthritis. Joint effusions, when present, are mildly inflammatory (leukocytes 3,000/μL, 80% mononuclear cells). Examination of synovial tissue specimens reveals synovial hyperplasia with a paucity of inflammation without granulomas. Neither articular nor bony lesions are seen on radiographs. Chronic sarcoid arthritis is polyarticular and may involve the same joints; but, unlike the acute situation, it is characterized by inflammatory synovial fluid (leukocytes 25,000/μL, 90% neutrophils), granulomas in synovial tissue specimens, and destructive bony lesions. Other musculoskeletal manifestations include acute or chronic monoarticular arthritis of the foot or wrist (uncommon); acute or chronic sarcoid myositis; and osseous sarcoidosis with "punched out" lytic lesions in the distal and middle phalanges. Muscle involvement in sarcoidosis is usually asymptomatic, yet at least 75% of such patients have noncaseating granulomas in muscle biopsy specimens.

The present patient had taken penicillin and oral contraceptive pills, either of which may be associated with erythema nodosum, but would not cause hilar adenopathy. As shown in the figure, there is enlargement of the hilar lymph nodes with no interstitial lung disease. An elevated level of angiotensin converting enzyme and a positive gallium scan are present in some patients with Löfgren's syndrome. Recurrent rheumatic fever was considered in this patient with fever, nodules, acute polyarthritis, and elevated acute-phase reactants. Unlike Löfgren's syndrome, the nodules of rheumatic fever are nontender, and the arthritis of rheumatic fever classically is migratory. Furthermore, this patient had no evidence of antecedent streptococcal infection, thus excluding acute rheumatic fever. Rheumatoid factor, although not present in this patient, is seen in up to 10% of sarcoid arthritis patients who may be misdiagnosed as rheumatoid arthritis. Prominent ankle involvement with periarthritis should suggest sarcoidosis. Complete resolution within 6 weeks is inconsistent with a diagnosis of rheumatoid arthritis and is generally the course with Löfgren's syndrome.

Löfgren's syndrome has an excellent prognosis, with a 90% remission rate. Most patients require only salicylates or other nonsteroidal anti-inflammatory drugs (NSAIDs). Occasional patients whose arthritis or erythema nodosum do not respond to NSAIDs may benefit from a short course of oral corticosteroids.

The present patient had a complete recovery and was treated symptomatically with nonsteroidal anti-inflammatory drugs.

Clinical Pearls

1. Löfgren's syndrome refers to the triad of acute polyarthritis, erythema nodosum, and hilar lymphadenopathy.

2. Nearly 50% of patients with Löfgren's syndrome have an acute self-limited form of sarcoidosis.

3. The HLA-B8,-DR3 haplotype may identify a group of sarcoidosis patients who are likely to have Löfgren's syndrome with complete recovery.

4. The synovitis of acute sarcoid arthritis with Löfgren's syndrome is less inflammatory than in chronic sarcoid arthritis, and synovial granulomas are not seen.

REFERENCES

1. Kaufman LD. Lofgren's syndrome (acute sarcoidosis) sine erythema nodosum mimicking acute rheumatoid arthritis. NY State J Med 1990;90:463–464.
2. Kellner H, Spathlling S, Herzer P. Ultrasound findings in Lofgren's syndrome: Is ankle swelling caused by arthritis, tenosynovitis or periarthritis? J Rheumatol 1992;19:38–41.
3. Mathur A, Kremer JM. Immunopathology, rheumatic features, and therapy of sarcoidosis. Curr Opin Rheumatol 1992;4:76–80.

PATIENT 12

A 54-year-old woman with muscle weakness and choking

A 54-year-old woman was transferred for evaluation of weakness. She was in good health, apart from a history of well-controlled hypertension, until 2 months prior to admission, when she noticed cold-induced blanching of her fingers. Subsequently, she developed difficulty arising from a sitting position and climbing stairs. She choked while eating and regurgitated both solids and liquids. Over the previous few days, she developed exertional dyspnea, but no cough. There was no arthritis, diplopia, paroxysmal nocturnal dyspnea, or edema.

Physical Examination: Temperature 98.0°; pulse 88, respirations 20; blood pressure 100/60. Skin: anterior chest telangiectases and thickening over the dorsal aspects of the MCP and PIP joints. Nailfold capillaroscopy: shown below. HEENT: no ptosis; gag reflex present but delayed. Chest: bibasilar crackles. Cardiac: normal. Abdomen: normal. Neurologic: proximal muscle weakness in both the upper and lower extremities; reflexes normal.

Laboratory Findings: WBC 10,800/μL with 65% neutrophils, 23% lymphocytes, 5% eosinophils, 7% monocytes; Hct 51%; ESR 8 mm/hr. Albumin 3.6 gm/dL, AST 157 IU/L, CPK 928 IU/L (10% MB isoenzyme), aldolase 48 IU/L. ANA 1:320 speckled. Chest radiograph: bibasilar fibrosis. Electromyography: insertional irritability and fibrillations consistent with myopathy. Forced vital capacity: 1.32 L. Barium swallow: hypofunction of pharyngeal muscles with dilatation and pooling in the piriform sinus and dysmotility of the upper third of the esophagus without aspiration. Biopsy of the left biceps muscle: degeneration and regeneration of fibers with interstitial accumulations of mononuclear cells; immunofluorescence showed IgG, IgM, and C3 in the interstitial areas.

Question: What is the diagnosis and cause of the patient's choking?

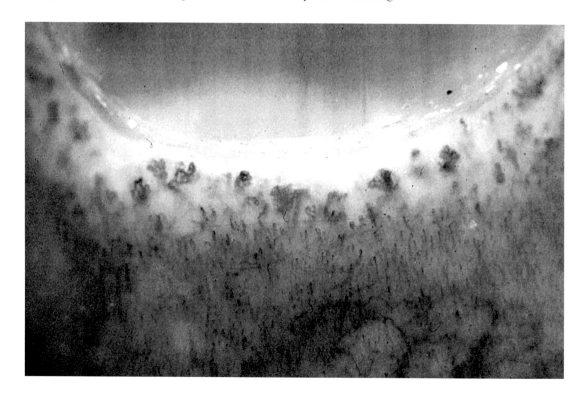

(provided by HR Maricq)

Diagnosis: Dermatomyositis with pharyngeal muscle involvement and pulmonary fibrosis.

Discussion: Inflammatory muscle diseases are classified by several types depending on the age of the patient, skin changes, associated diseases, and—more recently—the presence or absence of certain circulating antibodies. There are peaks of onset during childhood and again in later adult life. Inflammatory muscle diseases are relatively uncommon, occurring in only 5 to 10 per million population per year. The etiology remains unknown, but an association exists with malignancies in adults with these conditions.

Clinically, the onset of weakness is usually insidious and painless, although some patients may complain of achiness or actual pain. The weakness is almost exclusively of proximal musculature, and initially patients have difficulty performing tasks with arms raised and when rising from a seated position. Neck, respiratory, palatal, and pharyngeal muscles also can be involved, resulting in dysphonia, aspiration, and regurgitation.

Skin findings seen in dermatomyositis include the heliotrope rash on the upper eyelids, erythema of the "V" area of the anterior chest and the upper back (the so called "shawl sign"), and Gottron's papules over the proximal interphalangeal joints and metacarpophalangeal joints. Cracking of the skin of the distal fingers has been termed "mechanic's hands" and is seen most often in the antisynthetase syndromes. In these conditions, patients have serum antibodies to amino acid tRNA synthetases, such as the Jo-1 antigen, which is histidyl tRNA synthetase.

Pulmonary involvement can include hypoventilation due to respiratory muscle weakness, aspiration as a result of the pharyngeal muscle involvement, and interstitial fibrosis. The latter complication is associated with the presence of circulating antisynthetase antibodies such as Jo-1 antibodies. Cardiac muscle involvement rarely occurs but may lead to heart failure, conduction blocks, and arrhythmias. Elevation of the MB isoenzyme fraction does not necessarily indicate myocardial involvement because regenerating skeletal muscle also can make this isoenzyme.

The diagnosis of inflammatory muscle disease depends on the history, physical examination, and laboratory tests including muscle enzyme levels, electromyography, and muscle biopsy. Recently, magnetic resonance imaging, which shows bright areas in inflamed muscles, has been used to guide the biopsy location, but the expense of the procedure limits its general applicability. The differential diagnosis includes toxic myopathies, such as that induced by alcohol, disorders of the neuromuscular junction, such as myasthenia gravis, inherited muscular dystrophies, metabolic pathway disorders, such as McArdle's disease, and such infections as trichinosis. Nailfold capillaroscopy shows changes similar to those in scleroderma (dilated loops and avascular areas) and additional findings of branching capillary dilatations.

Electromyography shows insertional irritability (persistent spontaneous discharges after needle insertion), low amplitude polyphasic potentials, and fibrillations. The electromyogram can identify an appropriate muscle for biopsy; the biopsy should be performed on the contralateral noninstrumented muscle. Muscle biopsy demonstrates chronic inflammatory cells in perivascular and interstitial areas and both degeneration and regeneration of muscle fibrils. Dermatomyositis differs by including vessel-centered inflammation and deposition of immune complexes.

Treatment of inflammatory muscle disease involves the use of high-dose corticosteroids, e.g., prednisone 1 mg/kg/day orally. Physical activity should be limited initially, but progressive activity can be encouraged once improvement in strength occurs. The disease in some patients may be resistant to corticosteroids or may require such high doses that methotrexate or azathioprine must be added for their steroid-sparing effects.

The present patient demonstrated clinical and muscle histologic findings diagnostic of dermatomyositis. She was treated with prednisone, 60 mg per day, resulting in improvement of her proximal muscle strength but no change in her pharyngeal symptoms after several months of treatment. Methotrexate, 15 mg per week, was added, with resolution of her pharyngeal muscle weakness.

Clinical Pearls

1. Pulmonary involvement in patients with inflammatory myopathies may result from direct involvement of the respiratory muscles, from interstitial fibrosis, or from aspiration due to pharyngeal muscle weakness.

2. Both interstitial pulmonary fibrosis and the presence of "mechanic's hands" are seen in that subgroup of inflammatory muscle disease patients with circulating antibodies to RNA synthetases, the "anti-synthetase syndrome."

3. Treatment of inflammatory muscle disease includes daily oral corticosteroids, with addition of either methotrexate or azathioprine in those persons unresponsive or only partially responsive to corticosteroids.

4. Although disputed by some, there appears to be an association between adult inflammatory muscle diseases (particularly dermatomyositis) and malignancies.

REFERENCES

1. Cronin ME, Plotz PH. Current concepts in idiopathic inflammatory myopathies; polymyositis, dermatomyositis and related disorders. Ann Intern Med 1989;111:143–157.
2. Tazelaar HD, Viggiano RW, Pickersgill J, et al. Interstitial lung disease in polymyositis and dermatomyositis. Clinical features and prognosis as correlated with histologic findings. Am Rev Respir Dis 1990;141:727–733.
3. Love LA, Leff RL, Fraser DD, et al. A new approach to the classification of idiopathic inflammatory myopathy: myositis-specific autoantibodies define useful homogeneous patient groups. Medicine 1991;70:310–374.

PATIENT 13

A 12-year-old boy with juvenile rheumatoid arthritis and a swollen leg

A 12-year-old boy presented with a 1-week history of increased pain and swelling in his left knee and calf. He had juvenile rheumatoid arthritis beginning at 5 years of age, characterized by chronic pain and swelling and stiffness of the knees, wrists, and small joints of the hands. Rheumatoid factor and ANA were negative. Hemoglobin electrophoresis was normal. He responded to salicylates and did well until he recently developed increased pain and swelling of his left knee and calf.

Physical Examination: Temperature 100.3°. Extremities: warmth, tenderness, and pitting edema of the left knee and calf (see Figure). Left knee range of motion: 15 to 110°. Homan's sign positive, no crescent sign.

Laboratory Findings: Arthrocentesis (left knee): 45 mL sterile synovial fluid, leukocytes 11,055 cells/µL with 98% polymorphonuclear leukocytes and 2% monocytes. Doppler ultrasound: negative for deep venous thrombosis.

Question: What is the diagnosis?

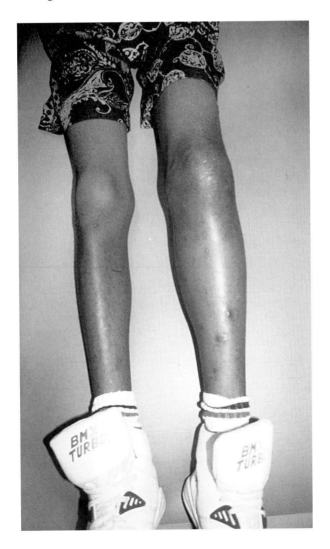

Diagnosis: Juvenile rheumatoid arthritis (JRA) with ruptured popliteal cyst.

Discussion: Juvenile rheumatoid arthritis, also termed juvenile arthritis or juvenile chronic arthritis, is the most common chronic rheumatic disease of childhood. Criteria proposed for the classification of JRA include: (1) onset before 16 years of age; (2) arthritis in one or more joints as defined by swelling or effusion or the presence of two or more of the following signs: limitation of range of motion, tenderness or pain on motion, and increased heat; (3) duration of disease of 6 weeks or longer; (4) distribution of articular complaints within the first 6 months of disease onset: (a) polyarthritis: five or more inflamed joints; (b) oligoarthritis: fewer than five inflamed joints; (c) systemic: arthritis with characteristic quotidian fever; (5) exclusion of other forms of juvenile arthritis. Among children with JRA, approximately 20% have systemic-onset, or Still's disease, with its characteristic quotidian fever and evanescent, salmon-pink macular rash. The polyarticular subset accounts for 40% of JRA cases, and the other 40% have an oligoarticular (pauciarticular) onset. Unlike adults with rheumatoid arthritis, most JRA patients (90%) are seronegative, i.e., they lack serum rheumatoid factor. JRA patients may have a positive ANA, particularly young girls in the pauciarticular subset who are at risk for chronic iridocyclitis.

Synovial outpouching is not uncommon in JRA, arising from the extensor hood of the proximal interphalangeal joints, wrists, or ankles. Whereas large synovial cysts, such as popliteal cysts, are common in adults with RA, they are rarely seen in JRA patients. Popliteal or Baker's cysts arise from the gastrocnemius semimembranosus bursa and communicate with the knee joint. Popliteal cysts may sometimes dissect or rupture into the calf, producing swelling and calf tenderness with a positive Homan's sign that resembles acute thrombophlebitis (*pseudothrombophlebitis*). The "hemorrhagic crescent sign" is a violaceous, crescent-shaped ecchymosis beneath one or both malleoli. It is seen in some, but not all, patients with rupture of a popliteal cyst. It is not seen in patients with deep vein thrombosis.

Popliteal cysts may be diagnosed either by ultrasonography or arthrography, but the latter is more sensitive for documenting rupture or dissection. Documentation is essential to avoid unnecessary anticoagulation, which might provoke bleeding into the cyst and soft tissues. It should be noted that in some patients dissected or ruptured popliteal cysts occur concomitant with deep vein thrombosis ("pseudo-pseudothrombophlebitis").

Only six cases of JRA complicated by ruptured popliteal cyst have been reported in the English literature. The present patient had recurrent knee effusions secondary to JRA and then presented with pseudothrombophlebitis. Deep vein thrombosis was excluded by ultrasonography, and a partially ruptured popliteal cyst was demonstrated by contrast arthrography. Treatment with bedrest, arthrocentesis, and intra-articular corticosteroids led to gradual resolution of the knee and leg swelling. Occasional patients with recurrent or refractory popliteal cysts may require surgical excision.

Clinical Pearls

1. JRA, the most frequent chronic rheumatic disorder of childhood, may be complicated by synovial cysts.

2. Popliteal cysts arising from the gastrocnemius semimembranosus bursa may rupture or dissect into the calf in adults with acute or chronic knee effusions, and rarely in children with JRA.

3. Dissection or rupture of a popliteal cyst causes calf pain and edema, and patients may have Homan's sign mimicking acute thrombophlebitis, i.e., *pseudothrombophlebitis.*

4. The hemorrhagic crescent sign beneath one or both malleoli is indicative of popliteal cyst rupture and helps distinguish it from acute thrombophlebitis.

REFERENCES

1. Kraag G, Thevathasan EM, Gordon DA, et al. The hemorrhagic crescent sign of acute synovial rupture. Ann Intern Med 1976;85:477–478.
2. Katz RS, Zizic TM, Arnold WP, et al. The pseudothrombophlebitis syndrome. Medicine (Baltimore) 1977;56:151–161.
3. Cassidy JT, Levinson, JE, Bass JC, et al. A study of classification criteria for a diagnosis of juvenile rheumatoid arthritis. Arthritis Rheum 1986;29:274–281.
4. Soslow AR. Popliteal cysts in a pediatric patient. Ann Emerg Med 1987;16:588–591.
5. Case records of the Massachusetts General Hospital. Weekly clinicopathological exercises. Case 17–1990. N Engl J Med 1990;322:1214–1223.

PATIENT 14

A 50-year-old woman with SLE, thrombocytopenia, and hip pain

A 50-year-old woman with systemic lupus erythematosus was treated for thrombocytopenia (platelet count 12,000/μL) with 60 mg per day of prednisone. Three weeks after starting corticosteroid she developed right groin pain that was exacerbated by weight bearing.

Physical Examination: Vital signs: normal. General: cushingoid appearance. Gait: antalgic. Hip: full range of motion.

Laboratory Findings: WBC 12,000/μL with 60% neutrophils, 33% lymphocytes, 5% monocytes; Hct 40%; platelet count 273,000/μL. ANA: 1:2560 homogeneous pattern. Anti-double-stranded DNA: 1:320. Lupus anticoagulant: negative. Anticardiolipin antibody: negative. Radiographs of hip: below.

Questions: What is the diagnosis and what course of action should be taken?

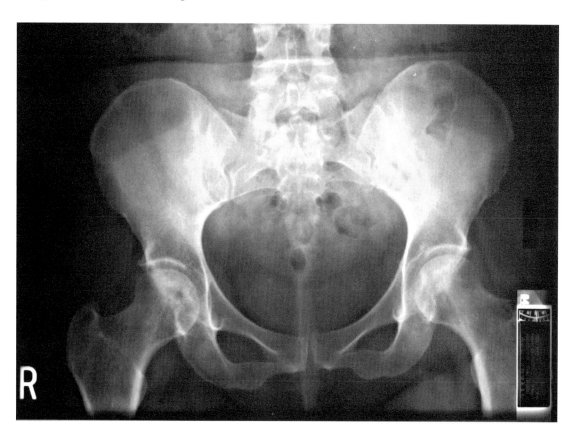

Diagnosis: Bilateral avascular necrosis of the femoral heads.

Discussion: Avascular (also known as ischemic, aseptic, or osteo-) necrosis of bone most commonly involves the femoral head, but the humeral head, the femoral condyles, and the proximal tibia also may be involved. Avascular necrosis may result from several causes but is most commonly seen in rheumatologic practice as a result of high-dose corticosteroid medication. Other causes include traumatic dislocations or femoral neck fractures and nontraumatic conditions such as alcohol abuse, sickle cell disease, decompression sickness, Gaucher's disease, and radiation. Whatever the cause, avascular necrosis results from impaired blood flow to the involved bone. In the femoral head, this impairment may be a result of arterial disruption after trauma or may be microvascular in nature. Because measurements of interosseous pressure in the latter type of avascular necrosis are elevated, it has been hypothesized that intramedullary pressure rises to a level that impedes blood flow. Increases in marrow fat, as seen in corticosteroid administration, result in such an increase in intramedullary pressure. This increase causes venous compression and stasis with eventual necrosis.

The occurrence of avascular necrosis during or after corticosteroid treatment is related to high doses. There appears to be a greater relationship to the peak corticosteroid dose than to the duration of therapy or to the cumulative dose.

The initial symptom of avascular necrosis of the femoral head is groin pain with intermittent radiation down the anteromedial thigh made worse by weight bearing. There is often night pain and morning stiffness. A sudden increase in pain may be noted when there is collapse of articular surface, and a distinct "clicking" associated with movement may be perceived. Range of motion of the hip early in avascular necrosis is not reduced, as the articular surfaces are not involved at that point.

Diagnosis of avascular necrosis requires a high index of suspicion. There is often a long delay between the onset of symptoms and radiographically evident changes, so that radiographs often show no changes at the time symptoms first appear. As the lesion develops, the radiographic appearance evolves through sclerosis to subchondral fracture (often evident as a "crescent sign" which appears as a thin line in the subchondral bone parallel to the articular surface) to collapse of the articular surface. When the initial radiographs are normal and avascular necrosis is suspected, bone scanning often shows either decreased uptake as a result of ischemia or "hot" areas due to the repair process. Because magnetic resonance imaging is very sensitive early in the course of necrosis and shows specific changes, it has become the method of choice for early detection. MRI scanning is often useful for examining the contralateral hip when avascular necrosis is radiographically evident in one hip.

Treatment of avascular necrosis of the hip has been somewhat controversial. Conservative treatment (avoiding weight bearing) is usually recommended, but is not often successful. Surgical treatment has taken two approaches. In hips that have not collapsed, core decompression may be applied, which involves removal of a core of cancellous bone from the ischemic segment. This decompresses the forces elevating the pressure in the femoral head. This technique is not always successful in preventing collapse. When collapse occurs, only femoral head replacement will eliminate the pain associated with the irregular joint space. If the process has not been longstanding, replacement of the acetabular component is not required, as this side of the joint is not involved in the process.

The present patient was treated with non-weight bearing, had some improvement in pain, and was to undergo core decompression in an attempt to salvage the native femoral head.

Clinical Pearls

1. Avascular necrosis of the hip may be traumatic in origin or the result of disruption of the microcirculation. This disruption is seen in sickle cell disease, alcoholism, Gaucher's disease, and with corticosteroid administration.

2. The occurrence of avascular necrosis in patients treated with corticosteroids is related to the peak dose of the medication rather than to the duration of the therapy or the cumulative dose. For this reason, steroids should always be prescribed at the lowest possible dose needed to treat the underlying condition.

3. When initially symptomatic, avascular necrosis of bone often is not apparent on radiographs. Magnetic resonance imaging is exquisitely sensitive and the diagnostic test of choice to diagnose early avascular necrosis.

4. Core decompression, in which a core of cancellous bone is removed from the femoral head, may help to avoid collapse of the bone. When collapse has occurred, only prosthetic replacement of the femoral head provides relief of symptoms.

REFERENCES

1. Zizic TM, Marcoux C, Hungerford DS, et al. Corticosteroid therapy asociated with ischemic necrosis of bone in systemic lupus erythematosus. Am J Med 1985;79:596–604.
2. Mitchell MD, Kundel HL, Steinberg ME, et al. Avascular necrosis of the hip: Comparison of MR, CT and scintigraphy. Am J Roentgenol 1986;147:67–71.
3. Steinberg ME, Corces A, Steinberg DR, et al. Osteonecrosis of the femoral head: Results of core decompression and grafting, with and without electrical stimulation. Clin Orthop Rel Res 1989;249:199–208.

PATIENT 15

A 28-year-old woman with left arm pain

A 28-year-old woman complained of diffuse pain of 3-months' duration affecting the left forearm and hand. During a hospital admission for management of an ovarian cyst, the patient's intravenous fluid infiltrated at the site of needle insertion in the left forearm. Subsequently, she developed persistent burning pain in the left arm and was referred for evaluation. There was no history of chest pain or dyspnea. Pain was made worse by movement, but she denied joint swelling, warmth, or erythema.

Physical Examination: Vital signs: normal. HEENT: normal. Chest: normal. Cardiac: normal. Abdomen: normal. Neurologic: exquisite tenderness to light touch of the left forearm and dorsum of the hand. Musculoskeletal: diffuse tenderness and 1+ edema of the left forearm; painful wrist with diminished flexion and extension; normal small joints of the left hand with full range of motion; decreased temperature of the left arm and hand with normal pulses.

Laboratory Findings: CBC: normal. Westergren ESR: 16 mm/hr. RF: negative. Thyroid function tests: normal. Hand radiographs: normal. Three-phase bone scan: see below.

Question: What is the diagnosis and recommended management?

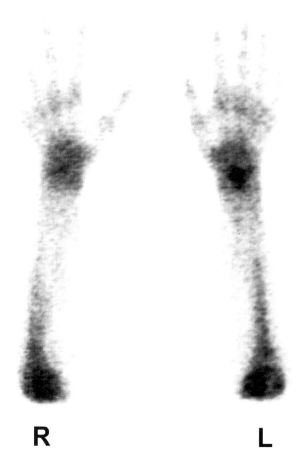

R   L

015

Diagnosis: Reflex sympathetic dystrophy syndrome.

Discussion: Reflex sympathetic dystrophy syndrome (RSDS) is a poorly understood condition characterized by severe pain affecting a distal extremity. Described initially by Silas Weir Mitchell, a surgeon operating on soldiers injured in the American Civil War, RSDS is the preferred term for conditions variably described as causalgia, Sudeck's atrophy, algoneurodystrophy, and shoulder-hand syndrome. The pain of RSDS is often described as burning in character. Diffuse tenderness frequently is accompanied by vasomotor changes (coolness, Raynaud's phenomenon, dusky hue), sudomotor changes (hyperhidrosis and hypertrichosis), and dystrophic skin changes (shiny skin with loss of wrinkling). Some patients complain that light touch triggers pain (*allodynia*), and some experience severe pain with repetitive mild or moderate stimuli (*hyperpathia*). These two symptoms, allodynia and hyperpathia, are considered to be diagnostic of RSDS, but neither is present in every case.

RSDS occurs equally in males and females. All age groups, including children, may be affected. Trauma is the most common precipitating event. Thrombophlebitis, as in the present case, and arterial thrombosis may be associated with the onset of RSDS. Myocardial ischemia, cerebrovascular accidents with hemiplegia, and peripheral nerve injuries are also associated with RSDS. In one-third of cases, there is no obvious precipitant.

In addition to soft tissue atrophy, bone atrophy may be evident. Radiologic changes are present in many patients, but plain radiographs may be normal early in the course of RSDS. Diffuse, patchy osteopenia is the most common abnormality on plain radiographs. The three-phase bone scan provides greater sensitivity and specificity in the diagnosis of RSDS. In up to 60% of cases, abnormalities are seen in each of the three phases: radionuclide blood flow phase, blood pool phase, and bone scan phase. In the present case, plain radiographs of the affected extremity were normal, yet the three-phase bone scan was abnormal (Figure), confirming the clinical diagnosis of RSDS. Recent studies suggest that dual x-ray absorptiometry is a sensitive indicator of bone loss that might be used to monitor response to treatment.

Successful treatment of RSDS often depends on early recognition and initiation of therapy. Exercises aimed at increasing the mobility of the affected extremity are the cornerstone of therapy. Pain control and efforts to interrupt the sympathetic nervous system are often utilized to facilitate maximal physical therapy. Pain may be diminished by the use of nonsteroidal anti-inflammatory drugs (NSAIDs), short-term narcotic analgesic drugs, topical capsaicin, and transcutaneous electrical nerve stimulator (TENS) units. For more aggressive treatment, paravertebral sympathetic blocks (e.g., stellate ganglion block), epidural blocks, or regional intravenous blocks (e.g., Bier block) may be employed. A brief course of high-dose prednisone may benefit some patients with RSDS. Intranasal administration of calcitonin has been shown to improve pain, range of motion, and work ability in some RSDS patients.

The present patient responded to a combination of physical therapy, NSAIDs, high-dose prednisone, and stellate ganglion blockade. A significant proportion of RSDS patients never fully recover and have chronic impairment of activities of daily living.

Clinical Pearls

1. The first classic description of what is now termed RSDS was reported in 1864, by the American Civil War surgeon Silas Weir Mitchell.

2. The presence of allodynia and/or hyperpathia are helpful clues to the diagnosis of RSDS in the patient complaining of diffuse extremity pain.

3. The three-phase bone scan provides greater diagnostic sensitivity and specificity than do plain radiographs.

4. Intranasal calcitonin may improve pain, range of motion, and work ability of some RSDS patients.

REFERENCES
1. Gobelet C, Waldburger M, Meier JL. The effect of adding calcitonin to physical treatment on reflex sympathetic dystrophy. Pain 1992;48:171–175.
2. Kozin F. Reflex sympathetic dystrophy syndrome: a review. Clin Exp Rheumatol 1992;10:401–409.
3. Inhofe PD, Garcia-Moral CA. Reflex sympathetic dystrophy. A review of the literature and a long-term outcome study. Orthop Rev 1994;23:655–661.
4. Arriagada M, Arinoviche R. X-ray bone densitometry in the diagnosis and followup of reflex sympathetic dystrophy syndrome. J Rheumatol 1994;21:498–500.

PATIENT 16

A 58-year-old woman with rheumatoid arthritis, fever, and dyspnea

A 58-year-old woman with rheumatoid arthritis had a 6-day history of anorexia and abdominal cramping with diarrhea and a 2-day history of fever, dyspnea, nonproductive cough, and headache. Her medications included prednisone (7.5 mg/day), methotrexate (20 mg/week), and hydroxychloroquine (200 mg bid).

Physical Examination: Temperature 101.3°; pulse 100; respirations 24; blood pressure 110/50. HEENT: white plaques on oral mucosa. Chest: crackles at both bases. Cardiac: tachycardia without murmurs or rubs. Abdomen: soft, nontender, with normal bowel sounds and no organomegaly. Extremities: synovitis of both wrists and ankles, no edema or cyanosis.

Laboratory Findings: Hct 41%; WBC 13,100/μL with 88% neutrophils, 10% lymphocytes, 2% monocytes, and no eosinophils. Blood chemistries: normal. ABG (room air): pH = 7.46, pO_2 60 mmHg, pCO_2 33 mmHg. Urinalysis: normal. Stool for WBCs: negative. Blood and sputum cultures: negative. Chest radiograph (below): bilateral basilar interstitial infiltrates with no effusions.

Questions: What are possible diagnoses and what course of action should be taken?

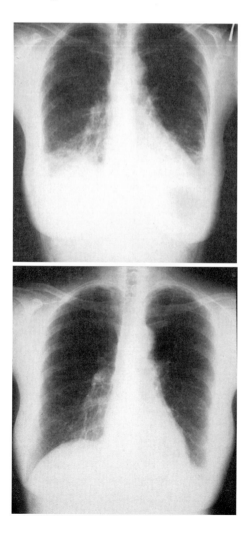

Diagnosis: Methotrexate pneumonitis.

Discussion: Although first reported in patients receiving high-dose methotrexate for leukemia, methotrexate pulmonary toxicity also may develop with the lower doses of the drug used to treat rheumatoid arthritis, polymyositis, or psoriasis. Among rheumatoid arthritis patients, the incidence of methotrexate lung toxicity ranges from 2% to 5%. The occurrence of methotrexate pneumonitis is not related to sex, age, dose, or duration of therapy, concomitant drug administration, or renal insufficiency. Stomatitis frequently accompanies lung toxicity. Studies differ as to whether underlying lung disease predisposes to methotrexate pneumonitis. The pathogenesis of this condition is unknown, but the observed histologic findings of mononuclear cells, giant cells, bronchiolitis, and fibrosis are consistent with a hypersensitivity reaction.

Pulmonary symptoms develop acutely, but headache and malaise may precede the development of nonproductive cough, dyspnea, and fever by several weeks. All of these symptoms may antedate radiographic lung involvement, which most commonly consists of bilateral interstitial infiltrates. Alveolar or nodular infiltrates, adenopathy, and effusions have also been reported. The white blood cell count is generally less than 15,000/μL, and eosinophilia is sometimes seen. Hypoxemia is usually present, and pulmonary function testing shows restriction.

Treatment of methotrexate pulmonary toxicity involves discontinuation of methotrexate, respiratory support, and administration of high-dose corticosteroids (1 mg prednisone/kg/d in divided doses). High-dose corticosteroid treatment has not been subjected to clinical trials in this condition, but its use appears justified considering the hypersensitive appearance of the pulmonary lesions. Most patients recover, although some may have residual restrictive lung disease. Some patients have had recurrence of pneumonitis when rechallenged with methotrexate, yet others have had methotrexate restarted without recurrence.

Because the clinical presentation of methotrexate pneumonitis typically resembles an infectious process, common pulmonary pathogens must be excluded before initiating steroid therapy. *Pneumocystis carinii* infection is a complication of methotrexate treatment of rheumatoid arthritis. This opportunistic infection closely resembles methotrexate lung toxicity, with fever, dyspnea, hypoxemia, and diffuse interstitial infiltrates on radiography. For this reason, bronchoscopy with special stains for pneumocystis and other potential pathogens should be performed when a patient presents with this constellation of signs and symptoms.

The present patient underwent bronchoscopy and bronchoalveolar lavage with cultures and stains for *Pneumocystis carinii* and *Legionella pneumophila,* as well as blood and urine cultures. The silver stain of the lung biopsy was negative, and treatment with intravenous methylprednisolone (15 mg every 6 hours) and erythromycin was initiated with substantial overnight improvement. All cultures and stains proved to be negative, and erythromycin was discontinued. Because fever and dyspnea recurred 2 days later when the prednisone dose was lowered to 20 mg/d, high doses were reinstituted with a slower taper. Chest radiograph findings resolved completely, and pulmonary function testing was normal 1 month later.

Clinical Pearls

1. Methotrexate pneumonitis is characterized by fever, dyspnea, nonproductive cough, hypoxemia, and diffuse interstitial infiltrates on chest radiography. Onset may be heralded by malaise and headache.

2. There is no association between methotrexate pneumonitis and drug dose or duration, age, sex, hematologic toxicity, concomitant drug administration, or renal insufficiency. There may be an association with underlying pulmonary disease or the occurrence of stomatitis.

3. Because methotrexate pneumonitis mimics infectious processes, pulmonary pathogens must be excluded when the patient is first evaluated. Of particular concern is *Pneumocystis carinii* pneumonia, which closely resembles methotrexate toxicity and has been reported to complicate methotrexate administration.

4. Treatment of methotrexate pneumonitis involves discontinuation of the offending medication, supportive respiratory care, and high doses of prednisone (0.5–1.0 mg/kg daily. Concomitant antibiotics may be needed pending results of cultures and stains.

REFERENCES

1. Ridley MG, Wolfe CS, Matthews JA. Life threatening acute pneuomonitis during low-dose methotrexate treatment for rheumatoid arthritis: a case report and review of the literature. Ann Rheum Dis 1988;47:784–788.
2. Leff RL, Case JP, McKenzie R. Rheumatoid arthritis, methotrexate therapy, and *Pneumocystis carinii* pneumonia. Ann Intern Med 1990;112:716.
3. Kremer JM, Phelps CT. Long-term prospective study of the use of methotrexate in the treatment of rheumatoid arthritis. Arthritis Rheum 1992;35:139–145.
4. Carroll GJ, Thomas R, Phatouros CC, et al. Incidence, prevalence, and possible risk factors for pneumonitis in patients with rheumatoid arthritis receiving methotrexate. J Rheum 1994; 21:51–54.
5. LeMense GP, Sahn SA. Opportunistic infection during treatment with low dose methotrexate. Am J Respir Crit Care Med 1994;150:258–260.
6. Golden M, Katz RS, Balk RA, et al. The relationship of preexisting lung disease to the development of methotrexate pneumonitis in patients with rheumatoid arthritis. J Rheumatol 1995;22:1043–1047.

PATIENT 17

A 50-year-old diabetic man with stiff hands

A 50-year-old man with longstanding insulin-dependent diabetes mellitus was referred for rheumatologic evaluation because of stiff hands. Over the past 5 years he had noted progressive stiffness of the joints of both hands, without pain, swelling, or warmth of the involved joints. His symptoms interfered with activities of daily living, including use of a syringe to withdraw and administer insulin. He had no other joint complaints except for mild pain and stiffness in both shoulders.

Physical Examination: Vital signs: normal. Skin: waxy thickening of skin over both hands without Raynaud's phenomenon or digital ulceration. HEENT: waxy-looking, hard exudates and microaneurysms in the fundi. Chest: normal. Cardiac: S4 gallop. Abdomen: normal. Neurologic: stocking-glove sensory neuropathy, negative Tinel's sign. Musculoskeletal: adhesive capsulitis affecting both shoulders, non-tender flexion contractures of multiple metacarpophalangeal and interphalangeal joints of the hands with no soft tissue or bony swelling (see below).

Laboratory Findings: CBC: normal. Fasting blood glucose: 215 mg/dL. Hemoglobin A_{1c}: 10%. Urinalysis: 1+ glucose and 1+ protein. Westergren ESR: 25 mm/hr. RF: negative. ANA: negative.

Question: What is the diagnosis?

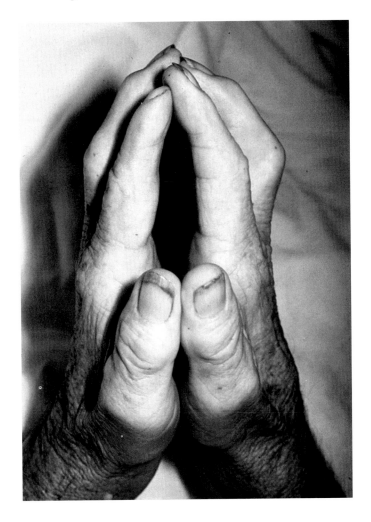

Diagnosis: Diabetic hand syndrome (diabetic cheiroarthropathy).

Discussion: Lundbaek first described a "diabetic hand syndrome" consisting of flexion contractures of the fingers and palmar skin thickening in five patients with long-standing diabetes mellitus. Other terms for the condition include the syndrome of limited joint mobility, the scleroderma-like syndrome of insulin-dependent diabetes mellitus, and diabetic cheiroarthropathy. "Cheiroarthropathy" comes from the Greek words *cheir* (hand), *arthron* (joint), and *pathos* (suffering), but this term is not entirely appropriate since the joint is involved only secondary to the collagenous changes of the skin and periarticular soft tissues. The syndrome occurs in diabetic children and adults. It is present in up to 50% of patients with insulin-dependent diabetes mellitus, and also occurs in non-insulin-dependent diabetic patients. The presence of flexion contractures affecting the interphalangeal and metacarpophalangeal joints correlates with the duration of diabetes, the degree of diabetic control, and the presence of microvascular disease, particularly retinopathy.

Patients with the diabetic hand syndrome present with painless, noninflammatory limitation of the hand joints. The condition typically begins in the fifth digit and extends radially, affecting the interphalangeal and metacarpophalangeal joints. Upon apposition of the hands, patients with the diabetic hand syndrome are unable to fully extend the MCP and PIP joints, giving rise to the "prayer sign" (see Figure). There is periarticular thickening of the skin, which assumes a waxy, tight appearance sometimes confused with scleroderma. Unlike scleroderma, the skin appendages are preserved, and patients lack features commonly seen in scleroderma, such as Raynaud's phenomenon, digital ulcers, and calcinosis.

Diabetes affects the hand in a number of other ways. Dupuytren's contractures are related to palmar fascial thickening and produce limited joint mobility, usually of the fourth and fifth fingers. Flexor tenosynovitis is quite common in diabetic patients, presenting as a painful trigger finger. Carpal tunnel syndrome is another common complication of diabetes, presenting as pain and numbness. Calcific shoulder periarthritis, like the diabetic hand syndrome, is correlated to the degree of diabetic control. It sometimes can be associated with reflex sympathetic dystrophy syndrome (RSDS) and may produce pain and limited motion of the hand (shoulder-hand syndrome). With the exception of Dupuytren's contractures, these other rheumatic manifestations are accompanied by pain in the hands and are easily distinguished from the diabetic hand syndrome.

The pathogenesis of the diabetic hand syndrome is believed to be related to glycation and nonenzymatic browning of dermal collagen. The level of hemoglobin A_{1c} appears to be related to joint contractures. Hyperglycemia is associated with increased glycation of collagen in diabetic patients. Glycation of human skin collagen is reduced significantly after several months of improved glycemic control. Glycemic control should be instituted and maintained to help prevent or reverse diabetic hand syndrome. Aldose reductase inhibitors have also been reported to improve the limited joint mobility of some patients with the syndrome.

This patient's glycemic control improved with closer monitoring of blood glucose and twice a day insulin administration. After 6 months, he noted less stiffness and increased hand joint mobility, and the hemoglobin A_{1c} fell toward normal levels.

Clinical Pearls

1. The diabetic hand syndrome, or diabetic cheiroarthropathy, is a common complication of diabetes related to increased glycation and nonenzymatic browning of skin collagen.

2. Limited joint mobility in a patient with diabetes mellitus indicates increased risk for microvascular disease, especially retinopathy.

3. Unlike most other diabetic complications affecting the hand, diabetic cheiroarthropathy is *painless.*

4. The *prayer sign* is a useful way to distinguish diabetic hand syndrome from other complications of diabetes affecting the hand.

REFERENCES

1. Starkman HS, Gleason RE, Rand LI, et al. Limited joint mobility (LJM) of the hand in patients with diabetes mellitus: relation to chronic complications. Ann Rheum Dis 1986;45:130–135.
2. McGuire JL. The endocrine system and connective tissue disorders. Bull Rheum Dis 1990;39:1–8.
3. Brik R, Berant M, Vardi P. The scleroderma-like syndrome of insulin-dependent diabetes mellitus. Diab Metab Rev 1991;7:121–128.
4. Lyons TJ, Bailie KE, Dyer DG, et al. Decrease in skin collagen glycation with improved glycemic control in patients with insulin-dependent diabetes mellitus. J Clin Invest 1991;87:1910–1915.

PATIENT 18

A 65-year-old woman with Raynaud's phenomenon and facial pain

A 65-year-old woman presented with a 1-year history of dysesthesia of the left side of the face with intraoral mucosal burning and numbness over the left zygoma. The burning was worsened by acidic, stringent, and solid foods. Difficulty eating and noxious taste to food led to a 23-pound weight loss. Three weeks ago, she noticed episodic blueness or whiteness of the fingertips upon exposure to cold. She had a history of chronic obstructive pulmonary disease with some dyspnea. There was no history of dysphagia, reflux esophagitis, dry eyes or mouth, diarrhea, skin changes, or muscle weakness.

Physical Examination: Vital signs: normal. HEENT: decreased sensation in the mandibular distribution of the left cranial nerve V; other cranial nerves normal. Skin: cyanosis of all fingers from PIP joints to tips; no sclerodactyly or digital pits.

Laboratory Findings: CBC, ESR, urinalysis, and renal function: normal. ANA: 1:320 with speckled pattern. Anti Scl-70: negative. Chest radiograph: normal. Brain MRI scan: normal except small cranial nerves V. Pulmonary function tests: consistent with small airways disease. Nailfold capillaroscopy: dilated capillary loops.

Question: What is the diagnosis?

Diagnosis: Systemic sclerosis *sine* scleroderma presenting as trigeminal neuralgia.

Discussion: Neurologic involvement in systemic sclerosis is quite unusual, occurring in less than 5% of cases. Trigeminal neuralgia in systemic sclerosis patients usually is associated with the limited cutaneous form (CREST syndrome), rather than with diffuse cutaneous systemic sclerosis. Nevertheless, trigeminal neuralgia occurs frequently enough to be considered a neurologic symptom secondary to systemic sclerosis. Features of an "overlap" syndrome with myositis, leukopenia, or Sjögren's syndrome are also common among scleroderma patients with trigeminal neuralgia. Many of those patients also demonstrate antibodies to U1 ribonucleoprotein. Trigeminal neuralgia usually occurs early in the course of systemic sclerosis, and, as in the present patient, may precede the diagnosis of the connective tissue disease.

Sensory changes may involve any or all divisions of the trigeminal nerve, with V2 and V3 more commonly involved. In about one-half of cases, the involvement is bilateral. Patients describe numbness, paresthesia, and either constant or episodic pain. Because sensation of intraoral structures is also innervated by the trigeminal nerve, patients may describe abnormal sensations within the mouth that may be intrepreted as alterations in taste. The pain may be described as burning or lancinating, and, when the latter is described, a trigger point may be identified. Initiation or exacerbation by such activities as chewing or tooth brushing is quite common. Because of the difficulty in chewing and recognizing particles in the mouth, difficult swallowing and coughing may occur.

The differential diagnosis of trigeminal neuralgia includes a number of conditions other than connective tissue diseases. Tumors, infections, and vascular abnormalities compressing the intracranial portions of the nerve cell all cause trigeminal neuralgia. Isolated trigeminal neuralgia is a diagnosis of exclusion and can be assured only by eliminating these other potential etiologies. CT or MRI scanning is useful in eliminating other potential etiologies.

The functional lesion appears to be in the peripheral course of the nerve as evidenced by the frequent separation of symptoms into those associated with distinct branches of the nerve. The pathologic lesion in trigeminal neuralgia complicating systemic sclerosis remains undefined but is likely to be vascular. Because trigeminal neuralgia is not associated with cases having extensive fibrotic skin disease, it is unlikely that fibrosis of the nerve from direct extension of cutaneous fibrosis is the cause.

Treatment of trigeminal neuralgia in systemic sclerosis does not differ from that of other causes, yet it is often very difficult to provide significant relief of symptoms. Oral amitriptyline or carbamazepine have been used with some success.

The present patient represents an unusual case in that she had no evidence of skin thickening either at the time of onset of the trigeminal neuralgia, nor did she have Raynaud's phenomenon initially. Her diagnosis of systemic sclerosis sine scleroderma was based on her Raynaud's phenomenon, positive ANA, and nailfold capillaroscopy. She was treated initially with amitriptyline without success and is currently taking carbamazepine with partial relief of her symptoms.

Clinical Pearls

1. Neurologic involvement in systemic sclerosis is unusual but includes involvement of the peripheral cranial nerve V, i.e., trigeminal neuralgia.

2. Trigeminal neuralgia in systemic sclerosis occurs more frequently in the limited cutaneous form (the CREST syndrome) than in the diffuse cutaneous form. Neuralgia may precede, coincide with, or follow the onset of symptoms of systemic sclerosis, but usually is not a late manifestation of the disease.

3. Symptoms of trigeminal neuralgia include facial and intraoral numbness, and burning or lancinating pain. Pain may be exacerbated by chewing or by brushing teeth, and a trigger point may be found on examination. The patient may describe taste disturbances, difficult swallowing, and cough.

4. The differential diagnosis of trigeminal neuralgia includes tumors, vascular causes, and infections. Imaging techniques (CT or MRI scanning) are necessary to exclude these causes.

5. Treatment of trigeminal neuralgia is difficult, but amitriptyline or carbamazepine have been used with some success.

REFERENCES

1. Teasdall RD, Frayha RA, Shulman LE. Cranial nerve involvement in systemic sclerosis (scleroderma): a report of 10 cases. Medicine (Baltimore) 1980;59:149–159.
2. Farrell DA, Medsger TA. Trigeminal neuropathy in progressive systemic sclerosis. Am J Med 1982;73:57–62.
3. Hietarinta M, Lassila O, Hietaharju A. Association of anti-U1RNP- and anti-Scl-70-antibodies with neurologic manifestations in systemic sclerosis. Scand J Rheumatol 1994;23:64–67.

PATIENT 19

A 65-year-old man with numbness of the left thigh

A 65-year-old man complained of numbness of the left thigh for the past 1 and one-half years. Initially, he noted a burning sensation that was intermittent, precipitated by walking and relieved by sitting. More recently, he noted constant numbness in the left anterior thigh that interfered with his ability to work as a tour guide. He complained of increased sensitivity to light touch in the same distribution as the numbness. He denied motor weakness, back pain, and constitutional symptoms. Past history was remarkable only for hypertension and benign prostatic hypertrophy.

Physical Examination: Temperature 98.6°; pulse 100; respirations 16; blood pressure 144/90; weight 227 pounds. Skin: normal. Lymph nodes: normal. HEENT: normal. Neck: enlarged thyroid without nodules. Chest: normal. Cardiovascular: normal. Abdomen: normal. Musculoskeletal: normal. Neurologic: CN II-XII normal, 5/5 strength in proximal and distal motor groups, DTR's 2+ and symmetric, diminished pinprick sensation over the anterolateral aspect of the left thigh (see Figure).

Laboratory Findings: CBC: normal. Westergren ESR: 10 mm/hr. Serum electrolytes: normal. Blood glucose: 93 mg/dL. Urinalysis: normal. T4: 6.19 µg/dL (4.50–12.00); TSH: 13.98 µl/mL (0.40–6.00).

Question: What is the diagnosis?

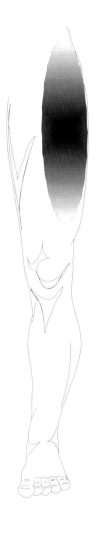

Diagnosis: Meralgia paresthetica and hypothyroidism.

Discussion: Meralgia paresthetica refers to a syndrome of pain or dysesthesia, or both, in the anterolateral thigh. It results from a peripheral neuropathy affecting the lateral femoral cutaneous nerve (L2–L3). The term **meralgia paresthetica** is derived from the Greek *meros,* thigh, and *algos,* pain. The lateral femoral cutaneous nerve is a sensory nerve that lies beneath the inguinal ligament just medial to the anterior superior iliac spine. Patients with meralgia paresthetica complain of intermittent burning pain associated with numbness and hypesthesia of the anterolateral thigh (see Figure). Motor function is not impaired, but symptoms are worsened by prolonged standing or walking.

Meralgia paresthetica usually arises from compression of the lateral femoral cutaneous nerve at the inguinal ligament, but sometimes may occur as a metabolic neuropathy, e.g., diabetes mellitus or hypothyroidism, in which case meralgia paresthetica may be the presenting feature. Compression of the lateral femoral cutaneous nerve at the inguinal ligament occurs most often due to obesity, but in some cases is due to compression from a corset, a belt worn too low ("Dunlap's disease"), abdominal distention from pregnancy or ascites, leg length discrepancy or, rarely, a tumor. Recently, meralgia paresthetica has been reported as a complication of a number of common surgical procedures, including laparoscopic inguinal herniorrhaphy, laparoscopic cholecystectomy, and coronary artery bypass, due to entrapment or compression of the nerve.

The diagnosis of meralgia paresthetica is based on the clinical finding of decreased sensation in the distribution of the lateral femoral cutaneous nerve (see Figure). Symptoms may be reproduced by pressing on the inguinal ligament just medial to the anterior superior iliac spine. Side-to-side comparison of sensory nerve conduction velocities or somatosensory evoked potentials may confirm the diagnosis in patients with unilateral meralgia paresthetica. The present patient had no response to electrical stimulation of the right lateral femoral cutaneous nerve.

Treatment of meralgia paresthetica involves the diagnosis and treatment of any underlying condition, such as diabetes or hypothyroidism; decompression of the nerve by avoidance of overly tight garments, or use of a heel lift to correct any leg-length discrepancy; or local corticosteroid injection. The vast majority of patients respond to conservative therapy. Intractable cases may respond to surgical neurolysis or sectioning of the lateral femoral cutaneous nerve.

The present patient improved when his hypothyroidism was treated.

Clinical Pearls

1. Meralgia paresthetica is a pure sensory neuropathy of the lateral femoral cutaneous nerve that presents as burning or numbness of the anterolateral thigh with normal motor function.

2. Although usually due to nerve compression at the inguinal ligament, meralgia paresthetica may be the initial manifestation of metabolic disease, e.g., diabetes mellitus or hypothyroidism.

3. Consider meralgia paresthetica in patients complaining of burning or numbness of the thigh after laparoscopic inguinal herniorrhaphy or other surgical procedures.

4. Meralgia paresthetica caused by lesions above the inguinal ligament carries a more serious prognosis than when lesions occur below.

REFERENCES
1. Suarez G, Sabin TD. Meralgia paresthetica and hypothyroidism. Ann Intern Med 1990;112:149.
2. Williams PH, Trzil KP. Management of meralgia paresthetica. J Neurosurg 1991;74:76–80.
3. Lagueny A, Deliac MM, Delliac P, et al. Diagnostic and prognostic value of electrophysiologic tests in meralgia paresthetica. Muscle Nerve 1991;14:51–56.
4. Regional Rheumatic Pain Syndromes. In Schumacher HR Jr (ed). Primer on the Rheumatic Diseases, 10th ed, Atlanta, GA, Arthritis Foundation, 1993, pp 283–284.

PATIENT 20

A 22-year-old woman with systemic lupus erythematosus
and dyspnea on exertion

A 22-year-old woman with a 10-year history of systemic lupus erythematosus (SLE) complained of dyspnea which, although chronic, had worsened over the past month. Two weeks previously a malar rash and pleuritic chest pain had recurred in association with right upper quadrant abdominal pain. Medications were hydroxychloroquine, 400 mg/d; prednisone 20 mg/d; and felodipine, 20 mg/d.

Physical Examination: Temperature 98.4°; pulse 110; respirations 26; blood pressure 140/98 with a 20 mmHg paradoxical pulse. Skin: malar rash. HEENT: several oral ulcers. Chest: clear. Cardiac: tachycardia, fixed splitting of S_2, no rub or murmur. Abdomen: normal bowel sounds, right upper quadrant tenderness, liver span 14 cm in the midclavicular line. Extremities: trace edema of lower extremities.

Laboratory Findings: WBC 9800/μL; Hct 43.1%; platelets 150,000/μL. Electrolytes, BUN, creatinine, and liver function tests: normal. Urinalysis: normal. PT and PTT: normal. VDRL: negative. Lupus anticoagulant: negative. Antiphospholipid antibodies: IgG positive. Antibodies to double-stranded DNA: positive at 1:80. Complement components: C3 50 mg/dL (86–184), C4 < 10 mg/dL. Chest radiograph: enlarged cardiac silhouette, small pleural effusions, clear lung fields. ECG: right axis deviation (R axis = 155°), right ventricular hypertrophy. ABG (room air): pH 7.48, pCO_2 32 mmHg, pO_2 78 mmHg. Spirometry: FVC 84% predicted. Single breath diffusion capacity: 74% predicted. Echocardiogram with Doppler study: moderate pericardial effusion, dilated right atrium and ventricle, peak right ventricular pressure estimate of 118 mmHg.

Question: What is the likely cause of the patient's dyspnea?

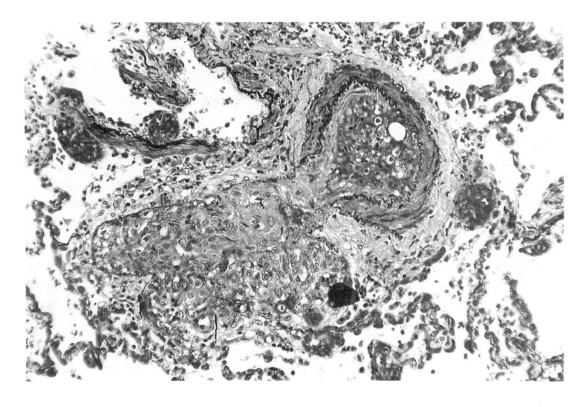

Diagnosis: Extensive plexogenic pulmonary arteriopathy secondary to SLE with antiphospholipid antibody syndrome (APS).

Discussion: The evaluation of dyspnea in a patient with SLE requires consideration of several possible causes including infection, drug toxicity, and extracellular volume overload, as well as direct effects of the disease itself. Cardiac involvment, including hypertension, occurs in 50 to 90% of SLE patients sometime during the course of their disease, and lung involvement occurs in 50 to 60%.

The most common involvement of the heart and lungs in SLE is serositis, with pleuritic or pericardial chest pain as the presenting symptom. Some pleural effusions are large enough to compromise ventilation, and pericardial effusions can cause tamponade, although this is a rare occurrence in SLE.

Pulmonary fibrosis does occur in SLE but is much less common than in systemic sclerosis. Dyspnea may be the initial pulmonary symptom. Chest radiography may be insensitive to changes severe enough to cause symptoms, and spirometry is more useful to uncover restrictive lung disease.

Pulmonary hypertension is not a common manifestation of SLE, occurring in only 5% of SLE patients in large series of patients. This phenomenon may occur secondary to interstitial fibrosis, chronic pulmonary emboli, or direct effects of a lupus anticoagulant on in situ thrombosis in pulmonary arterioles. Either a lupus anticoagulant (antiphospholipid antibody; see Patient 6) or a deficiency of antithrombin III as a result of renal disease with nephrotic syndrome increases the risk of pulmonary emboli in SLE patients. Emboli can be large and cause acute symptoms, or small and chronic, resulting in pulmonary hypertension.

When pulmonary hypertension is discovered in an SLE patient, one should attempt to identify the underlying cause. Ventilation/perfusion scanning to look for emboli, heart catheterization to evaluate for left heart failure (as a possible cause of right heart failure), and Doppler studies of the venous systems of the lower extremities should be performed. Tests for lupus anticoagulant, antiphospholipid antibodies, and antithrombin III deficiency are also appropriate.

Treatment of pulmonary hypertension associated with the lupus anticoagulant and/or antiphospholipid antibodies should include anticoagulation to prevent future emboli. Supplemental oxygen can improve dyspnea and reduce pulmonary vascular resistance. Vasodilators (hydralazine or calcium channel blockers) are usually ineffective over the long term, but may have acute effects in lowering pulmonary artery pressure.

In the present case, dyspnea and chest pain had prompted a ventilation lung scan several years earlier that was normal. The patient died suddenly in the hospital after experiencing increased dyspnea following Valsalva manuever. Autopsy findings included extensive plexiform arteriopathy with occlusion of vessels by proliferation of endothelial cells (see Figure). Bronchial arteries communicated with distal pulmonary arteries and supplied blood to the pulmonary capillaries. No nephritis was found.

Clinical Pearls

1. Chest pain and dyspnea in a patient with SLE must prompt a search for causes related to the disease itself (serositis, parenchymal fibrosis, pulmonary hypertension, and others), infection (including opportunistic infections), and pulmonary emboli.

2. SLE patients are at increased risk of pulmonary emboli due to several factors, including loss of antithrombin III as a result of nephrosis, the presence of a lupus anticoagulant, and being bedridden.

3. Pulmonary hypertension in SLE may develop for one of several reasons, including chronic pulmonary emboli or the development of plexogenic arteriopathy. Both of these have been associated with the presence of a lupus anticogulant or antiphospholipid antibodies.

4. Treatment of pulmonary hypertension in SLE (as in all other conditions) is problematic but should include chronic anticoagulation and supplemental oxygen if the patient is hypoxemic.

REFERENCES

1. Hughson MD, McCarty GA, Brumback RA. Spectrum of vascular pathology affecting patients with the antiphospholipid syndrome. Hum Pathol 1995;26:716–724.
2. Bick RL, Ancypa D. The antiphospholipid and thrombosis (APL-T) syndromes. Clinical and laboratory correlates. Clin Lab Med 1995;15:63–84.
3. Hellman DB, Kirsch CM, Whiting-O'Keefe Q, et al. Dyspnea in ambulatory patients with SLE: prevalence, severity, and correlation with incremental exercise testing. J Rheumatol 1995;22:455–461.

PATIENT 21

A 55-year-old man with weight loss, pain, and swollen extremities

A 55-year-old man presented with a several months' history of swelling of the arms and legs accompanied by pain in the wrist, knee, and ankle joints. He had no prior history of arthritis. His limb pain was associated with a 30-pound weight loss and generalized weakness. He smoked cigarettes but denied cough, dyspnea, or chest pain.

Physical Examination: Temperature 100.1°; pulse 112; respirations 16; blood pressure 140/80. Skin: normal. Lymph nodes: normal. HEENT: normal. Neck: normal. Lungs: normal. Cardiovascular: II/VI systolic ejection murmur. Abdomen: normal. Neurologic: normal. Extremities: 2+ bilateral pitting edema to the knees; exquisite bilateral tenderness over the tibia and radius; moderate-sized warm effusions in the ankles, knees, and wrists, with full range of motion. Clubbing of the fingers and toes was present.

Laboratory Findings: WBC 6,400/µL, Hct 32.5%, platelets 598,000/µL. Serum electrolytes: normal. Urinalysis: normal. Chest radiograph: 5-cm diameter nodule in the posterior segment of the right lower lobe. ECG: normal. Synovial fluid analysis: clear, yellow fluid, leukocytes 1000 cells/µL with 20% neutrophils, 20% lymphocytes, and 60% monocytes; normal Gram stain; no crystals by polarized light microscopy. Arm radiographs: see below.

Course: A transbronchial lung biopsy was performed.

Question: What is the cause of this man's limb pain?

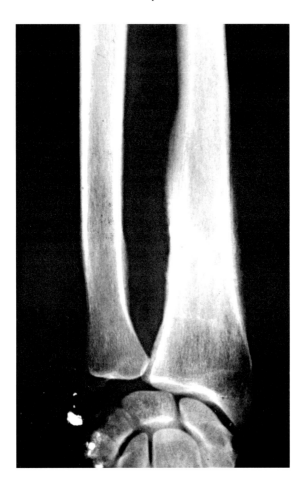

Diagnosis: Hypertrophic osteoarthropathy (HOA) secondary to carcinoma of the lung.

Discussion: Hypertrophic osteoarthropathy (HOA) refers to the presence of digital clubbing in association with periostosis of the long bones. HOA may occur as a primary disease process, or it may occur secondary to a variety of underlying conditions. Primary HOA is a rare autosomal dominant condition, also known as *pachydermoperiostosis,* in which finger clubbing and periostosis occur in association with variable skin changes of pachydermia, seborrhea and folliculitis. Far more common is the secondary form of HOA, in which clubbing and periostosis occur in association with an underlying disease. Secondary HOA may occasionally be *localized,* for example due to patent ductus arteriosus, infective arterial graft, aneurysm, or hemiplegia. Usually, secondary HOA is *generalized* and occurs in association with underlying pulmonary, cardiac, hepatic, or intestinal disease. Bronchogenic carcinoma, which was diagnosed in the present patient, is perhaps the most common pulmonary cause of HOA, but HOA also may be seen in patients with metastatic or other forms of lung cancer, cystic fibrosis, chronic lung infections or pulmonary fibrosis. The most common cardiac cause of HOA is congenital cyanotic heart disease. HOA is also seen in patients with infective endocarditis (SBE). Diseases of the gastrointestinal tract including hepatic cirrhosis, carcinoma, and inflammatory bowel disease are other secondary causes of HOA. A thorough search for an underlying illness should be undertaken in any patient presenting with new-onset HOA.

Although some patients may be asymptomatic, others complain of severe pain in the bones, particularly the arms and legs. As in the present patient, patients with malignant lung tumors may present with incapacitating limb pain and joint swelling. Clubbing is usually evident in the fingers and sometimes in the toes. Careful physical examination reveals the site of greatest tenderness to be periarticular, along the shaft of the radius, tibia or fibula. The ankles, knees and wrists are the joints most commonly affected by pain, swelling, and warmth. There is usu-

ally full range of motion, and joint contractures are rare. Synovial effusions are relatively noninflammatory. Synovial biopsy specimens show little or no inflammation but marked vascular changes including congestion and platelet fibrin thrombi.

The diagnosis of HOA rests with the clinical observation of digital clubbing in association with periostosis. Although periostosis may be suspected by eliciting pain on palpation of the long bones, it is usually diagnosed by plain radiographs of tubular bones showing periosteal proliferation with preservation of the joint space (see Figure). Radionuclide bone scans are very sensitive indicators of periostosis but are rarely required to establish the diagnosis of HOA.

Little evidence exists to support the once popular neurogenic theory of HOA. The pathogenesis of HOA more likely involves proliferation of dermal and periosteal fibroblasts under the influence of various growth factors. One theory suggests that megakaryocytes or large platelets, which normally are trapped and fragment within the pulmonary capillary bed, escape to the systemic circulation via right-to-left shunts. These thrombocytes then impact and fragment distally, releasing granules containing growth factors, e.g., platelet-derived growth factor (PDGF). The formation of platelet clumps on infected heart valves, aneurysms or infected grafts could lead to a similar phenomenon in patients with HOA in whom right-to-left shunts are not present. PDGF is a potent mitogen and chemoattractant for fibroblasts and smooth muscle cells whose release might stimulate mesenchymal cell growth, leading to clubbing and periostosis.

Salicylates and other NSAIDs may provide partial relief of symptoms in some patients with secondary HOA. Treatment of the underlying condition may provide dramatic but often temporary improvement. For example, HOA may resolve following treatment of infective endocarditis or subside following resection of a lung tumor. The present patient's lung tumor was unresectable and symptoms of HOA persisted until death.

Clinical Pearls

1. Hypertrophic osteoarthropathy (HOA) is a clinical syndrome of digital clubbing and periostosis due to excessive proliferation of dermal and periosteal fibroblasts.

2. Patients with HOA secondary to lung cancer may present with incapacitating limb pain, whereas patients with comparable HOA secondary to cyanotic congenital heart disease may be asymptomatic.

3. Synovial fluid from joints affected by HOA is typically thick, yellow and noninflammatory.

4. The megakaryocyte/platelet clump hypothesis can account for virtually all cases of secondary HOA.

REFERENCES

1. Schumacher HR Jr. Hypertrophic osteoarthropathy: rheumatologic manifestations. Clin Exp Rheumatol 1992;10(S-7):35–40.
2. Martinez-Lavin M. Pathogenesis of hypertrophic osteoarthropathy. Clin Exp Rheumatol 1992;10(S-7):49–50.
3. Dickinson CJ. The aetiology of clubbing and hypertrophic osteoarthropathy. Eur J Clin Invest 1993;23:330–338.

PATIENT 22

A 64-year-old woman with generalized musculoskeletal pain, difficulty sleeping, and weight loss

A 64-year-old woman presented with difficulty sleeping, weight loss, and diffuse pain in her jaw, neck, head, shoulders, hands, back, legs, and toes. She denied joint swelling and muscle weakness, but complained of prolonged morning stiffness. There had been no changes in her vision, but her jaw hurt when she chewed. She had lost 16 pounds over the previous 2 months and noted afternoon temperature elevations to 100.3°. She had taken trazodone nightly during the last 10 years with good response for a diagnosis of fibromyalgia.

Physical Examination: Temperature 99.2°; pulse 82; respiration 18; blood pressure 100/70; weight 132 pounds. General: elderly, tearful woman. HEENT: mild temporal tenderness. Chest, cardiac, abdomen: normal. Musculoskeletal: normal muscle strength, diminished neck rotation; shoulder abduction painful to 90°; other joints normal; tenderness over paraspinal muscles of neck and lumbar area, trapezius muscles, deltoid insertions, and greater trochanters.

Laboratory Findings (2 months before evaluation): WBC 6400/μL; Hct 40%; platelets 187,000/μL; Westergren ESR 7 mm/hr; electrolytes normal; creatinine 0.9 mg/dL; liver function tests normal; thyroid stimulating hormone <0.1 U/mL (normal 0.4 to 6.0); thyroxine 12.71 μg/dL (normal 4.5 to 11.5) CK 35 IU/L. Temporal artery biopsy (see Figure).

Questions: What is the differential diagnosis and what tests should be ordered?

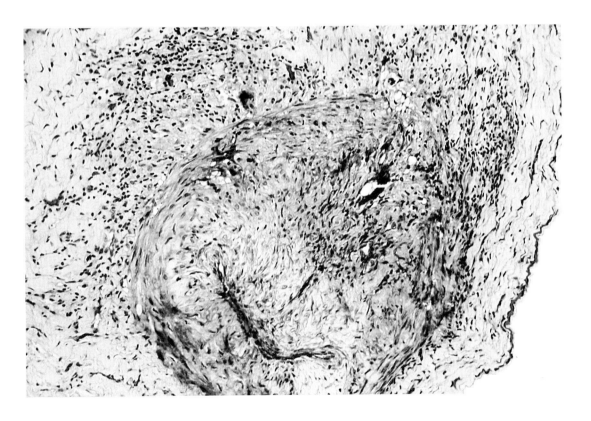

Diagnosis: Temporal arteritis and fibromyalgia.

Discussion: Evaluation of a patient with nonspecific achiness requires consideration of a wide range of rheumatic, malignant, metabolic, and psychiatric diseases. Complete physical examination (including pelvic and breast examinations), basic laboratory testing such as CBC, sedimentation rate, electrolytes, serum calcium, liver function tests, thyroid function tests, and routine health maintenance screening (mammography, Pap smears, prostate exams, and PSA) often give clues to the diagnosis.

Depression often presents as diffuse musculoskeletal complaints without physical findings. Associated symptoms include feelings of worthlessness, crying, anorexia, sleep disturbances, and suicidal thoughts. Fibromyalgia is characterized by generalized pain and tenderness at characteristic locations: posterior base of the skull, cervical paraspinal muscles, trapezius muscles, lateral humeral epicondyles, pectoralis muscles lateral to the second costochondral junction, upper gluteal area, greater trochanter, anserine bursae, and the junction of the Achilles tendon and gastrocnemius muscle. Fibromyalgia patients complain of difficulty falling asleep or frequent awakening, feeling unrested in the morning, and easy fatigue. Except for various tender points the physical examination as well as the laboratory evaluation is usually normal.

Malignancy can present with generalized pain that is usually severe and accompanied by abnormal levels of serum calcium or alkaline phosphatase; radiographs may show blastic or lytic bony lesions. Bone scans may demonstrate neoplastic lesions. Inflammatory muscle disease presents as proximal muscle weakness that is usually painless, but can include myalgia. Elevated serum creatine kinase and abnormal EMG confirm the diagnosis.

Hypothyroidism can cause muscle pain and stiffness and, although creatine kinase levels may be elevated, there is little weakness. Hyperthyroidism can result in painless proximal muscle weakness with normal serum muscle enzyme levels.

Polymyalgia rheumatica is a syndrome of pain and stiffness in the shoulder and pelvic girdle areas. Patients complain of neck and low back pain. Morning stiffness is a prominent symptom. Temporal arteritis (a giant cell arteritis of the external cephalic circulation) can occur either alone or with polymyalgia rheumatica. Symptoms include weight loss, low grade fever, temporal headache, jaw claudication (tiring of the masseter muscle with chewing), and visual disturbances ranging from diplopia or blurring to sudden and irreversible monocular blindness. Polymyalgia rheumatica and temporal arteritis occur in persons over 50 years of age. Laboratory findings include elevated ESR and anemia. There are often no physical findings, although the temporal arteries may be tender and/or enlarged. In cases where temporal arteritis is suspected, biopsy of the temporal artery may demonstrate giant cell inflammation centered at the internal elastic lamina. Treatment of polymyalgia rheumatica and temporal arteritis involves the use of steroids. With polymyalgia alone, prednisone doses of 10 to 20 mg/day generally provide relief within a few days. Temporal arteritis requires higher prednisone doses (1 mg/kg/day).

In the present patient, laboratory testing showed a Westergren ESR of 106 mm/hr. Liver and thyroid function tests were normal, as was the CK. Temporal artery biopsy showed classic changes of giant cell arteritis. Treatment with prednisone, 60 mg/day, resulted in prompt normalization of the ESR. After 18 months of treatment and weaning of prednisone to 5 mg/day, ESR was normal and weight had returned to baseline. She continued to have generalized muscle aches and tender points consistent with fibromyalgia.

Clinical Pearls

1. Generalized somatic complaints may be due to one of several inflammatory, metabolic, malignant, or psychiatric illnesses.

2. While inflammatory myopathies may cause myalgia, pain is usually overshadowed by proximal muscle weakness.

3. Thyroid disease may present with musculoskeletal symptoms. In hyperthyroidism, proximal muscle weakness without pain or elevations of muscle enzymes occurs. In hypothyroidism, muscles are stiff and painful and, although serum muscle enzymes may be elevated, weakness does not occur.

4. Polymyalgia rheumatica occurs in persons over 50 years old and is characterized by stiffness in the shoulder and pelvic girdle areas. An associated syndrome, temporal arteritis, is characterized by constitutional symptoms, headache, jaw claudication, and ocular ischemia. Both are associated with elevated sedimentation rates and responsiveness to oral corticosteroids.

5. Depression can present as diffuse musculoskeletal complaints, sleep disorders, and weight loss.

REFERENCES

1. Hunder GG, Bloch DA, Michel BA, et al. The American College of Rheumatology 1990 criteria for the classification of giant cell arteritis. Arthritis Rheum 1990;33:1122–1128.
2. Goldenberg DL. Psychiatric and psychologic aspects of fibromyalgia syndrome. Rheum Dis Clin North Am 1989;15:105–113.
3. Dorwart BB. Arthropathies associated with endocrine diseases. In Schumacher HR Jr (ed). Primer on the Rheumatic Diseases, 10th ed. Atlanta, Arthritis Foundation, 1993, pp 242–244.
4. Cimmino MA, Salvarani C. Polymyalgia rheumatica and giant cell arteritis. Bailliere's Clin Rheumatol 1995;9:515–527.
5. Sandler NA, Ziccardi V, Ochs M. Differential diagnosis of jaw pain in the elderly. J Am Dent Assoc 1995;126:1263–1272.

PATIENT 23

A 37-year-old physician with acute polyarthritis

A 37-year-old physician presented in March with a 1-day history of polyarthritis involving the hands, wrists, elbows, and knees. She had been in excellent health until 2 weeks earlier, when she developed low-grade fever, headache, and myalgia followed 1 week later by an erythematous eruption on her legs and a sore throat. There was no improvement after a 5-day course of oral penicillin. Two weeks before the onset of the present illness, she was exposed to a child with fever and a facial rash characterized by bright red cheeks. Her past medical history was remarkable for hepatitis B infection 10 years earlier.

Physical Examination: Temperature 99.5°; respirations 20; heart rate 88; blood pressure 112/70. Skin: faintly erythematous, macular eruption over the legs. Nodes: normal. HEENT: normal. Lungs: normal. Cardiac: II/VI systolic ejection murmur. Abdomen: normal. Neurologic: normal. Musculoskeletal: symmetric synovitis involving the PIP and MCP joints of the hands and moderate-sized, warm effusions of the knees with full range of motion.

Laboratory Findings: WBC 10,700/μL with 70% neutrophils, 15% lymphocytes, 12% monocytes and 3% eosinophils; Hct 29.8% with normal RBC indices; platelets 326,000/μL. Serum chemistries: normal. Westergren ESR: 42 mm/hr. Rheumatoid factor: negative. ANA: negative. ASO titer: negative. Viral serologies were obtained.

Question: What is the most likely cause of this patient's acute polyarthritis?

Diagnosis: Acute parvovirus B19-associated arthritis.

Discussion: Human parvovirus B19 is the etiologic agent of the common childhood illness erythema infectiosum, or *fifth disease* (historically named for its classification as the fifth of six childhood exanthems). In recent years human parvovirus B19 has been recognized as a frequent cause of acute polyarthritis in adults.

Most cases of erythema infectiosum occur in the spring in children of primary school age. The illness may be sporadic or epidemic. Parvovirus B19 is a small, single-stranded DNA virus usually transmitted by nasal secretions. Transmission may also occur, however, from transfusion of infected blood. The average incubation period is 7 days and ranges from 4 to 16 days. In children, the disease is characterized by red cheeks that look as if they have been slapped, and a blotchy macular eruption on the trunk and extremities. Erythema infectiosum is very common, with up to 60% of adults having serologic evidence (IgG antibodies) of past infection.

Rheumatic manifestations of erythema infectiosum are uncommon in children. Only 10% of infected children have arthralgia, and even fewer have arthritis. Rarely, children develop a chronic arthritis resembling juvenile chronic arthritis. In adults, particularly women, parvovirus B19 infection is accompanied by joint symptoms in the majority of cases. Arthralgia or arthritis is polyarticular and symmetric, in a distribution similar to that of rheumatoid arthritis, i.e., MCP, MTP, PIP, wrist, ankle and knee joints. Joint symptoms are self-limited and resolve completely by 2 weeks in the majority of patients. Some patients may have chronic or intermittent joint symptoms, but erosive joint disease does not occur. Tests for rheumatoid factor and ANA are usually negative but may be tran-siently positive in some patients. Evidence for persistence of B19 virus or B19 DNA sequences exists in patients with chronic parvoviral arthropathy, as well as in some patients with acute but nonchronic arthropathy.

The characteristic facial rash of childhood erythema infectiosum is usually lacking in adults. Adults and children may have a subtle reticular rash on the trunk or extremities. Some adults experience flu-like symptoms such as headache, myalgia, and low-grade fever. Mild transient anemia may occur in the viremic phase. In patients with underlying chronic hemolytic anemia, parvovirus infection may precipitate aplastic crisis. Infection in immunocompromised patients may result in severe, persistent anemia.

Although adult parvovirus arthropathy may mimic RA, rheumatoid factor is usually absent and the illness is self-limited. Other considerations in a patient with acute polyarthritis include rubella and hepatitis viral infections and Lyme disease. These conditions can be distinguished from parvovirus infection by serologic testing. IgM antibodies against human parvovirus B19 may be present for 2 to 3 months. IgG antibodies are present in up to 60% of adults, prevalent enough to be of no diagnostic use.

The present patient was treated with aspirin, three tablets qid, for 2 weeks. The joint pain and swelling resolved and did not recur when aspirin was discontinued. Six weeks after presentation she was asymptomatic, the ESR was normal and the Hct was 35.7%. She had been exposed to a child with erythema infectiosum, had a self-limited acute polyarthritis, and had serologic evidence of acute infection, i.e., the presence of IgM antibodies against parvovirus B19.

Clinical Pearls

1. Consider parvovirus B19 infection (erythema infectiosum) in an adult with acute, symmetric polyarthritis associated with flu-like symptoms and skin rash.

2. Confirm the diagnosis with serologic tests for anti-B19 IgM antibody.

3. Women are more likely to have arthritis with acute parvovirus infection than are men or children; parvovirus B19 infection may account for as many as 12% of all cases of acute polyarthralgia or polyarthritis in adults.

4. Mild transient anemia may occur in cases of parvovirus B19 arthropathy.

REFERENCES

1. Foto F, Sang KG, Scharosch LL, et al. Parvovirus B19 specific DNA in bone marrow from B19 arthropathy patients: evidence for B19 virus persistence. J Infect Dis 1993;167:744–748.
2. Naides SJ. Infectious arthritis. B. Viral and less common agents. In Schumacher HR Jr (ed). Primer on the Rheumatic Diseases, 10th ed. Atlanta, Arthritis Foundation, 1993, pp 198–201.
3. Marshall JB, McMurray R. Acute polyarthritis. Fifth disease passed from child to adult. Postgrad Med 1994;95:165–168.

PATIENT 24

A 44-year-old woman with a history of proteinuria presents with urinary retention

A 44-year-old woman with a 3-year history of proteinuria (membranous glomerulonephritis by biopsy), negative ANA, and discoid lupus erythematosus was treated with trimethoprim/sulfamethoxazole for complaints of difficulty in urination. Over several days she developed low-grade fever, posterior headache accompanied by posterior cervical pain, difficulty arising from a chair, and greater difficulty voiding.

Physical Examination: Temperature 101.3°, pulse 98, respirations 28, blood pressure 120/80 mmHg. Skin: no alopecia or rash. ENT: no oral ulcers. Chest: clear. Heart: normal. Abdomen: palpable urinary bladder. Joints: without arthritis. Neurologic: fully oriented; normal cranial nerves and upper extremities; lower extremities with diminished strength (2/5); 2+ patellar and achilles reflexes; bilateral Babinski signs; a T_4 sensory level.

Laboratory Findings: WBC 12,100/μL; Hct 33%; platelet count 222,000/μL. Electrolytes, BUN and creatinine: normal. Urinalysis: normal. RPR: negative. ANA 1:80, anti-double-stranded DNA 1:10, anti-Smith and anti-RNP antibodies negative. C3 81.5 (low), C4 14.3 (low). ESR: 72 mm/hr. Antiphospholipid antibodies and lupus anticoagulant: negative. CSF analysis: protein 196 mg/dL; WBC 109/μL (50% neutrophils, 14% lymphocytes, 36% macrophages); RBC 1,024/μL; India ink stain: negative; routine and AFB smears and cultures: negative. Spinal MRI (shown): expansion of the cervical and thoracic spinal cord with intense diffuse heterogeneous enhancement of cord with gadolinium.

Question: What is the diagnosis and treatment?

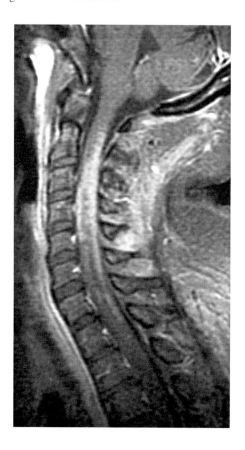

Diagnosis: Transverse myelitis secondary to systemic lupus erythematosus.

Discussion: About 25% of patients with SLE have involvement of the central or peripheral nervous systems. Neuropsychiatric SLE may have protean manifestations, including seizures, psychosis, dementia, movement disorders, cerebrovascular occlusions, aseptic meningitis, peripheral neuropathies, myositis, and transverse myelitis. Myelitis is a rare manifestation, occurring in less than 1% of SLE patients.

CNS infections are more likely to occur in immunocompromised patients and must always be considered a cause of nervous system symptoms and signs in patients with SLE. Bacterial meningitis or mycobacterial or fungal infections may occur in the CNS, usually as a result of spread from a non-CNS focus. Herpes simplex, disseminated Varicella zoster, and cytomegalovirus infection are more likely to occur in immunocompromised hosts.

Some medications have CNS effects that must be considered when a patient presents with CNS signs and symptoms. Ibuprofen and trimethoprim/sulfamethoxazole each have been associated with aseptic meningitis in SLE patients. Corticosteroids (particularly in high daily doses) may cause profound personality changes similar to mania or psychosis with hallucinations, insomnia, and pressured speech.

Transverse myelopathy may result from herniated nucleus pulposus, epidural infection or bleeding, metastases, tuberculosis, syphilis, vasculitis, and viral infections (HIV, polio virus, herpes zoster, rabies). Characteristic symptoms are urinary retention and lower extremity weakness and sensory loss. When the upper cord is affected, quadriaplegia including respiratory compromise may occur.

Transverse myelitis usually occurs in a patient with known SLE, but rarely may be the presenting manifestation. At autopsy the pathology varies from necrotizing vasculitis of the anterior spinal arteries and its branches to bland thrombotic occlusion of the vessel. No single laboratory test is diagnostic of transverse myelitis, but CSF pleocytosis and elevated protein with a low glucose level are characteristic. Antiphospholipid antibodies and/or a lupus anticoagulant are sometimes present. MRI scanning has dramatically improved the likelihood of diagnostic confirmations and should be performed quickly.

Treatment with high-dose corticosteroids should be initiated immediately, with 1 gm methylprednisolone intravenously every day for 3 days (pulse therapy) followed by prednisone at 1 mg/kg/day. Intravenous cyclophosphamide should be given at 0.5 to 1 gm/m^2 body surface area. Treatment should be prolonged since many patients have had long recovery intervals.

The present patient was treated as above and was admitted to the rehabilitation service. When discharged 5 weeks later she was able to use her right arm. High-dose oral prednisone and monthly intravenous cyclophosphamide were continued. Eight months later she regained bladder function, 1 year later she was walking with a walker, and 2 years later she was completely recovered and had returned to work.

Clinical Pearls

1. Nervous system involvement in SLE may include psychosis, depression, dementia, seizures, movement disorders, cerebrovascular occlusion, myelopathy, and peripheral neuropathy.

2. Transverse myelitis in SLE can involve any part of the spinal cord and rarely may be the presenting manifestation of SLE.

3. Cerebrospinal fluid usually shows a pleocytosis, elevated protein, and low glucose.

4. When transverse myelitis is suspected, an MRI scan of the spinal cord should be performed as soon as possible to confirm the diagnosis and exclude other causes.

5. Immunosuppressive treatment of transverse myelitis in SLE should be aggressive and prolonged, including high-dose corticosteroids and intravenous cyclophosphamide.

REFERENCES

1. Harisdangkul V, Doorenbos D, Subramony SH. Lupus transverse myelopathy: better outcome with early recognition and aggressive high-dose intravenous corticosteroid pulse treatment. J Neurol 1995;242:326–331.
2. Lopez-Dupla M, Khamashta MA, Sanchez AD, et al. Transverse myelitis as a first manifestation of systemic lupus erythematosus: a case report. Lupus 1995;4:239–242.
3. Neuwelt CM, Lacks S, Kaye BR, et al. Role of intravenous cyclophosphamide in the treatment of severe neuropsychiatric systemic lupus erythematosus. Am J Med 1995; 98:32–41.

PATIENT 25

A six-year-old boy with neck pain

A six-year-old boy presented with a 6-month history of torticollis. His parents reported that the patient had intermittent neck pain over the preceding 2 years, but did not seem to experience any other articular complaints. There was no history of head or neck trauma. The family history was negative for arthritis.

Physical Examination: Vital signs: normal. Skin: normal. Lymph nodes: normal. HEENT: normal. Neck: no masses or goiter; no tenderness or tightness of the sternocleidomastoid muscles. Back: nontender. Neurologic: normal. Musculoskeletal: Cervical spine was nontender; head was rotated 45 degrees to the left and tilted toward the right; range of motion testing showed inability to extend the neck, head rotation to neutral on the right and full on the left; right knee had small warm effusion with a 10° flexion contracture.

Laboratory Findings: CBC: normal. Serum chemistries: normal. Urinalysis: normal. Westergren ESR: 46 mm/hr. RF: negative. ANA: positive at 1:640, with speckled pattern. HLA B-27: negative. CT scan: soft tissue density surrounding the odontoid process with 8 mm anterior subluxation of C1 on C2; rotation of C1 to the left with complete subluxation of the right lateral mass of C1 anterior to the lateral mass of C2 (see below).

Questions: What is the underlying diagnosis and what is the cause of this patient's torticollis?

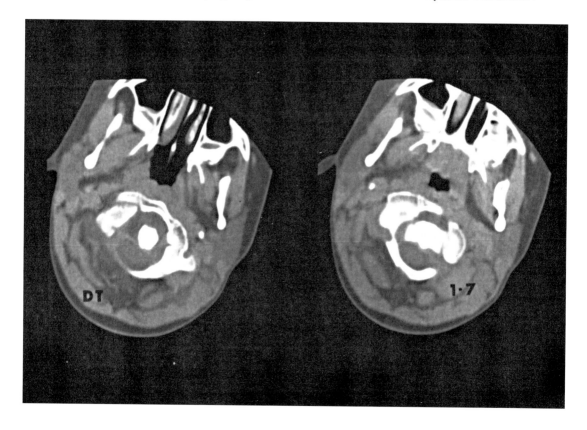

Diagnosis: Pauciarticular JRA with anterior and rotatory subluxation of C1 on C2.

Discussion: Juvenile chronic arthritis (juvenile rheumatoid arthritis, JRA) is the most common chronic rheumatic disease of childhood. JRA has been divided into three major subsets based on the number of joints affected during the first 6 months of disease, as well as the presence or absence of characteristic systemic features: *polyarticular* (five or more joints), *pauciarticular* (four or fewer joints) and *systemic* (intermittent fever, rash, hepatosplenomegaly, lymphadenopathy and arthritis). Pauciarticular disease accounts for 50% of all cases of JRA and usually involves the knees, ankles or elbows, in descending order of frequency. Young children with pauciarticular JRA, particularly those with a positive ANA, are at risk for chronic anterior uveitis and must be monitored by routine slit lamp examinations.

The cervical spine is rarely the presenting joint (<3% of all cases), yet up to 70% of children with JRA have radiographic evidence of cervical spine involvement at some point in the course of their disease. Neither severe neck pain nor torticollis are frequent complaints, and the presence of either should alert the clinician to possible intercurrent conditions, such as fracture or infection. Torticollis has rarely been reported to be the presenting manifestation of JRA. More frequently, the child with JRA and cervical spine involvement is found to have peripheral joint disease and painless loss of motion of the cervical spine. Children with polyarticular or systemic-onset JRA are more likely to have cervical spine involvement than are children with pauciarticular-onset JRA.

In either adults or children with chronic synovitis, cervical spine disease can involve the atlantoaxial joint and/or the subaxial spine may be involved. Radiographic surveys of children with JRA demonstrate anterior atlanto-axial subluxation in up to 20% of cases. Anterior subluxation of C1 on C2 is present in children when the distance between the posterior aspect of the ring of C1 and the anterior margin of the odontoid process of C2 measured in flexion exceeds 4.5 mm (as compared to 3 mm in adults). Extreme subluxation may produce compression myelopathy, but this is rarer in JRA than in adults with RA. Several cases of myelopathy due to atlanto-axial subluxation have been reported in children who had both JRA and Down syndrome.

Rotatory subluxation of C1 on C2 occurs far less commonly, in either children with JRA or adults with RA, than does anterior atlanto-axial subluxation. Laxity of the C1–C2 apophyseal joint capsules may permit lateral and rotatory subluxation. Unilateral collapse of the lateral mass of C1 and/or C2 may also occur. This complication results in nonreducible rotational head tilt. It should be suspected in the patient with neck pain, crepitus, fixed head tilt deformity, and rotational deformity. In patients with nonreducible rotational head tilt, the tilt is always toward the most affected side.

Radiographic changes in the subaxial cervical spine are also seen in children with JRA. Zygapophyseal joint fusion is seen most frequently, reported to be present in 25% to 50% of patients with the disease. Spontaneous fusion occurs initially in the posterior elements and later may involve the vertebral bodies and disc spaces. Growth disturbance of the vertebral bodies and disc spaces follows zygapophyseal joint fusion. Subaxial subluxation is a much less common finding in JRA patients than in adults with RA.

The present patient was treated initially with nonsteroidal anti-inflammatory drugs, physical therapy, external traction, and a halo vest. One year later, at age 7, he developed synovitis in the other knee and increased left rotation of the head. He was placed in halo traction once again, with reduction of the anterior subluxation to 4 mm and improvement in the head tilt. After 3 months, he was placed in a cervical brace to maintain the head in the midline. Serial radiographs demonstrated spontaneous osseous fusion of C1 and C2 anteriorly and at the right lateral mass, as well as fusion at the zygapophyseal joints from C1 to T2. At age 7 and one-half, he was noted to have nongranulomatous anterior uveitis on routine slit lamp examination. The uveitis resolved with topical steroid and cycloplegic eyedrops and no loss of visual acuity occurred. At age 15, he was asymptomatic with normal visual acuity, a residual 5-degree flexion contracture of the right knee, and complete fusion of the cervical spine.

Clinical Pearls

1. Pauciarticular-onset is the most common subset of JRA. Patients who are ANA-positive are at risk for chronic anterior uveitis.

2. Arthritis affecting the cervical spine is rarely the presenting manifestation of JRA (<3% of cases), but ultimately the majority of patients will have limited motion and/or radiographic abnormalities.

3. Atlanto-axial subluxation is present when the atlanto-dens interval exceeds 4.5 mm in children, as compared to 3.0 mm in adults.

4. Neurologic deficits from atlanto-axial subluxation are rarely seen in children with JRA but have been reported in a number of children with both JRA and Down syndrome.

5. Nonreducible rotational head tilt occurs due to rotatory subluxation of C1 on C2, or collapse of the lateral mass, and the head always tilts toward the involved side.

REFERENCES

1. Halla JT, Fallahi S, Hardin JG. Nonreducible rotational head tilt and atlantoaxial lateral mass collapse. Clinical and roentgenographic features in patients with juvenile rheumatoid arthritis and ankylosing spondylitis. Arch Intern Med 1983;143:471–474.
2. Hensigner RN, DeVito PD, Ragsdale CG. Changes in the cervical spine in juvenile rheumatoid arthritis. J Bone Joint Surg 1986;68-A:189–198.
3. Espada G, Babini JC, Maldonado-Cocco JA, et al. Radiologic review: the cervical spine in juvenile rheumatoid arthritis. Semin Arthritis Rheum 1988;17:185–195.

PATIENT 26

A 47-year-old woman with rash and muscle weakness

A 47-year-old woman with silicone breast implants for 5 years developed a rash on her hands and neck, myalgia, profound weakness, and dysphagia. She had recently been treated for a urinary tract infection, but was on no medication when the rash and weakness developed.

Physical examination: Temperature 97.8°; pulse 110; respirations 20; blood pressure 110/70. Skin: purplish discoloration of eyelids, periungual infarcts, Gottron papules over MCP and PIP joints, erythematous rash in "V" of neck. Lymph nodes: none palpable. Chest: clear. Heart: normal. Breasts: implants symmetric nontender, no discharge. Abdomen: no organomegaly. Pelvic examination: normal. Extremities: normal. Neurologic: hoarse voice, weak gag reflex. Musculoskeletal: motor strength of proximal upper and lower extremities 0/5, distal 3/5.

Laboratory tests: WBC 21,800/μL with 98% neutrophils, 2% lymphocytes; Hct 34%; platelets 314,000/μL. Electrolytes normal. BUN 8 mg/dL, creatinine 0.4 mg/dL. Chest radiograph: normal. ECG: sinus tachycardia. Urinalysis: normal. SGOT 357 IU/L, albumin 2.1 gm/dL. CPK 5829 IU/L, MM fraction 98.8%. Muscle biopsy: focal necrosis and acute mild inflammation by neutrophils and eosinophils. Skin biopsy (neck): interface dermatitis and mucin. Pap smear: normal. Abdominal CT scan: normal.

Questions: What are the diagnostic possibilities and which tests would you order?

Diagnosis: Dermatomyositis associated with ovarian cancer.

Discussion: Poly/dermatomyositis is an idiopathic inflammatory process producing proximal muscle weakness. Other causes of proximal muscle weakness are glucocorticoid excess (either as result of tumor or iatrogenic administration), myasthenia gravis, Eaton-Lambert syndrome, disorders of lipid metabolism (such as carnitine palmityltransferase deficiency), hypophosphatemia, hyperthyroidism, and exposure to a number of toxic substances.

Poly/dermatomyositis is the most commonly seen inflammatory cause of proximal muscle weakness. Inflammatory myopathy may also occur in patients with connective tissue diseases, such as systemic lupus erythematosus or systemic sclerosis (scleroderma). In poly/dermatomyositis, proximal muscle weakness is greater than distal muscle involvement. The occurrence of skin changes distinguish poly- from dermatomyositis. In dermatomyositis, the characteristic skin eruptions include a heliotrope rash (purplish discoloration) of the eyelids, erythema in the anterior "V" of the neck, erythema over the neck and shoulders posteriorly (the "shawl" sign), and Gottron papules over the extensor surfaces, e.g., the MCP and IP joints. Patients may complain of dysphagia due to pharyngeal muscle weakness and dyspnea due to respiratory muscle weakness.

Inflammatory myopathies are unusual diseases, with an incidence of 2 to 10 cases per million. The association of myositis with malignancy has been a topic of controversy for many years. Most evidence points to a link between myositis and malignancy in adults, more so for dermatomyositis than for polymyositis. Malignancies associated with myositis mirror those occurring in the general population. Ovarian cancer may be over-represented in women with dermatomyositis. Most commonly myositis is diagnosed within a year of detecting a malignancy.

Screening for malignancy in patients with myositis need not be complicated by expensive and invasive tests. Mammography, stool guaiac tests, Pap smears, rectal examination, and chest radiography are indicated, in addition to follow-up of any leads from a thorough history and physical examination.

Laboratory findings in both poly- and dermatomyositis include elevated muscle enzymes (CPK, aldolase, SGOT, LDH), relatively small increases in erythrocyte sedimentation rate and, in some patients, myoglobinuria. Electromyography (EMG) shows fibrillation potentials, short duration, low amplitude, complex (polyphasic) action potentials. Electromyography can help one decide which muscle to biopsy. A muscle contralateral to one showing electrical abnormalities should be chosen to give the highest chance of obtaining histologic confirmation of the diagnosis. Recently, MRI scanning of muscles has been used to identify areas of inflammation and can help to pinpoint biopsy sites. Biopsied muscle shows chronic inflammatory cells in the perivascular and interstitial areas, predominantly lymphocytes but also macrophages, plasma cells, neutrophils, and eosinophils.

Silicone breast implants have been implicated as possible causes of connective tissue diseases including poly/dermatomyositis, but the evidence is conflicting. Large epidemiologic studies do not support a relationship between silicone implants and such illnesses.

In the present case, there was an initial response to high-dose corticosteroids and intramuscular methotrexate, standard treatments for myositis. However, within 2 months she developed increasing abdominal girth due to ascites. Pelvic ultrasonography revealed an ovarian mass which on biopsy proved to be adenocarcinoma. She died 4 months later of metastatic ovarian carcinoma.

Clinical Pearls

1. Proximal muscle weakness accompanied by a skin eruption is most commonly due to dermatomyositis, but systemic lupus erythematosus and systemic sclerosis (scleroderma) may also be complicated by inflammatory muscle disease.

2. In controlled epidemiologic studies reported to date, there appears to be no link between silicone breast implants and the development of connective tissue diseases, including poly/dermatomyositis.

3. There is a link between malignancy and inflammatory muscle disease in adults but not in children.

4. Tumors associated with poly/dermatomyositis are those that occur commonly in the general population (lung, stomach, pancreas, ovarian, colon, renal).

5. In most cases of myositis associated with malignancy, the diagnosis of myositis precedes that of malignancy (paraneoplastic syndrome), usually by less than 1 year. Treatment of the underlying malignancy may result in improvement or remission of the myositis.

REFERENCES

1. Callen JP. Myositis and malignancy. Curr Opin Rheumatol 1994;6:590–594.
2. Zantos D, Zhang Y, Felson D. The overall and temporal association of cancer with polymyositis and dermatomyositis. J Rheumatol 1994;21:1855–1859.
3. Whitmore SE, Rosenshein NB, Provost TT. Ovarian cancer in patients with dermatomyositis. Medicine 1994;73:153–160.
4. Airio A, Pukkala E, Isomaki H. Elevated cancer incidence in patients with dermatomyositis: a population based study. J Rheumatol 1995;22:1300–1303.

PATIENT 27

A 22-year-old man with cold intolerance, muscle weakness, and fatigue

A 22-year-old man was referred for evaluation of cold intolerance and muscle fatigue. He complained of generalized arthralgia on exposure to cold, but denied pallor or cyanosis of the digits. He complained of generalized muscle weakness, fatigue, and a tremor affecting the hands. At age 10, a subcutaneous mass measuring 5 cm × 2 cm × 1 cm was excised from the right upper leg, and the pathology specimen was read as osteoid metaplasia. His past history was otherwise remarkable only for childhood otitis media and sinusitis. A brother had diabetes mellitus and CREST syndrome.

Physical Examination: Temperature 97.2°; heart rate 72; respirations 16; blood pressure 100/64. General appearance: short stature with round face. HEENT: normal. Neurologic: mild mental retardation; Chvostek sign and Trousseau sign were present, as well as a fine intention tremor. Musculoskeletal: small hands and feet with normal joints; normal strength. Extremities: no Raynaud's phenomenon, clubbing, or edema.

Laboratory Findings: CBC: normal. Na^+ 141 mEq/L; K^+ 4.6 mEq/L; Cl^- 101 mEq/L; HCO_3^- 27 mEq/L; BUN 12; creatinine 1.0 mg/dL; calcium 6.2 mg/dL; phosphorus 7.9 mg/dL; alkaline phosphatase 168 IU/L; glucose 84 mg/dL; albumin 4.5 g/dL; AST 18 IU/L; uric acid 2.0 mg/dL; cholesterol 142 mg/dL; total bilirubin 0.7 mg/dL; total protein 7.5 g/dL; LDH 112 IU/L. Urinalysis: normal. PTH 1373 pg/mL (normal 50–330 pg/mL). T4 4.28 µg/dL (4.5–12.0 µg/dL); TSH 13.9 µ/mL (0.4–6.0 µu/mL). Hand radiographs: see below.

Question: What is the diagnosis?

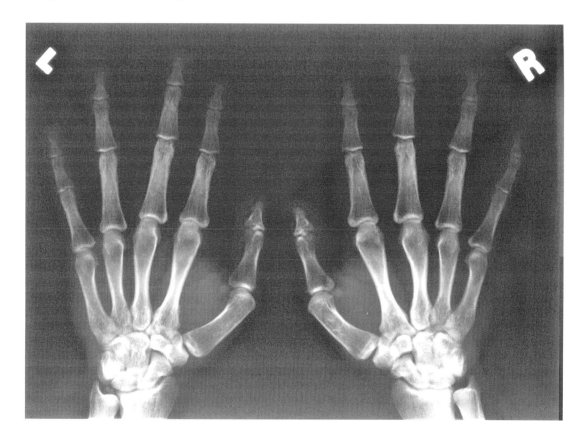

Diagnosis: Pseudohypoparathyroidism type Ia (Albright's hereditary osteodystrophy).

Discussion: Hypocalcemia, whether due to primary hypoparathyroidism or pseudohypoparathyroidism, may result in a variety of musculoskeletal signs and symptoms, including muscle weakness and fatigue. In primary hypoparathyroidism there is inadequate secretion and low serum levels of parathyroid hormone (PTH), either due to aplasia of the glands (e.g., DiGeorge syndrome) or surgical removal of the glands. In pseudohypoparathyroidism, the glands are present, serum levels of PTH are high, but there is end-organ resistance to the action of PTH.

There are at least two distinct forms of pseudohypoparathyroidism. In type Ia, also known as Albright's hereditary osteodystrophy, hormonal resistance is not limited to PTH, and there is a constellation of abnormal features such as short stature, variable mental retardation, brachydactyly, and ectopic ossification. The present patient had each of these features, together with hypocalcemia, hypophosphatemia, elevated PTH levels and hypothyroidism. His initial manifestation was subcutaneous ossification at age 10, but the diagnosis was not made until 12 years later. Other common sites of calcification and ossification are the basal ganglia and the paraspinal ligaments.

A characteristic skeletal change of pseudohypothyroidism is shortening of the metacarpals and metatarsals, especially the fourth. The foreshortened fourth metacarpal produces the "knuckle, knuckle, dimple, knuckle" sign when viewing the clenched fist. A radiographic clue for pseudohypoparathyroidism is a positive metacarpal sign: normally a line drawn tangential to the heads of the fourth and fifth metacarpals does not intersect the third metacarpal or just contacts its distal aspect. In pseudohypoparathyroidism, such a line may intersect the third metacarpal, indicating disproportionate shortening of the fourth and fifth metacarpals. This sign is neither specific nor particularly sensitive, since it is seen in other conditions and may not be noted in some patients with pseudohypoparathyroidism where the third metacarpal is also shortened (as in the present case).

In type Ib pseudohypoparathyroidism, the patient's physical appearance is normal and hormonal resistance is limited to PTH. In another variant of Albright's hereditary osteodystrophy, termed pseudopseudohypoparathyroidism, patients have the physical features but lack the hormone resistance of type Ia patients.

The end-organ resistance in type Ia pseudohypoparathyroidism is due to a deficiency in the cell membrane-associated guanine nucleotide regulatory protein (G-unit). The G proteins are a family of guanine nucleotide-binding proteins that mediate signal transduction across cell membranes and have a heterotrimeric structure composed of α, β, and γ subunits. Albright's hereditary osteodystrophy is an autosomal dominant condition in which there is reduced expression or function of the α subunit of the stimulatory G protein ($G_s\alpha$) of adenylate cyclase. This protein is required for the action of PTH and other hormones that use cyclic AMP as the intracellular second messenger. In some patients, the disease is caused by single-base substitutions in the $G_s\alpha$ gene and is due to inherited mutations in this G protein. As in the present patient, primary hypothyroidism is commonly seen in patients with pseudohypoparathyroidism type Ia, perhaps due to the same deficiency in G-protein function leading to resistance to TSH.

The present patient was treated with calcium supplements, Vitamin D (50,000 units/day), and synthroid, 0.1 mg/day. On this regimen the calcium and phosphorus normalized (9.3 mg/dL and 3.0 mg/dL, respectively), as did the T4 and TSH (6.58 μg/ml and 1.55 μu/mL, respectively). His cold intolerance, muscle weakness and fatigue resolved.

Clinical Pearls

1. Albright's hereditary osteodystrophy is an autosomal dominant syndrome characterized by short stature, variable mental retardation, brachydactyly, ectopic calcifications, and frequently pseudohypoparathyroidism.

2. The routine examination of the clenched fist may suggest Albright's hereditary osteodystrophy: the foreshortened fourth metacarpal produces the so-called "knuckle, knuckle, dimple, knuckle" sign.

3. Subcutaneous calcification or ossification may be the presenting manifestation of pseudohypoparathyroidism Ia or pseudopseudohypoparathyroidism.

4. End-organ resistance to PTH and other hormones in patients with pseudohypoparathyroidism results from a mutation in the α subunit of the G-protein leading to altered signal transduction.

REFERENCES

1. Resnick D, Niwayama G. Parathyroid disorders and renal osteodystrophy. In Resnick D, Niwayama G (eds). Diagnosis of Bone and Joint Disorders, 2d ed. Philadelphia, WB Saunders, 1988, pp 2219–2285.
2. McGuire JL. The endocrine system and connective tissue disorders. Bull Rheum Dis 1990;39:1–8.
3. Patten JL, Johns DR, Valle D, et al. Mutation in the gene encoding the stimulatory G protein of adenylate cyclase in Albright's hereditary osteodystrophy. N Engl J Med 1990;322:1412–1419.

PATIENT 28

A 22-year-old bone marrow transplant recipient with skin thickening

A 22-year-old woman was referred for evaluation of skin thickening. Four years earlier she received a bone marrow transplant (BMT) for treatment of chronic myelogenous leukemia (CML). She had two episodes of acute graft-versus-host disease with mucositis and skin rash that responded to cyclosporin A therapy. Fifteen months after the BMT she noted pruritus and thickening of the skin over the abdomen that progressed to involve the skin over the shoulders. She denied symptoms of Raynaud's phenomenon, gastroesophageal reflux, or dyspnea.

Physical Examination: Vital signs: normal. Skin: ivory-colored plaques of sclerotic skin over each shoulder and lichenification of skin over the abdomen. HEENT: xerostomia without parotid gland enlargement or mucosal lesions. Chest: normal. Cardiac: normal. Abdomen: normal. Neurologic: normal. Musculoskeletal: normal. Extremities: no acrosclerosis, cyanosis, or edema.

Laboratory Findings: CBC: normal. ESR: 20 mm/hr. Serum chemistries: normal. Liver panel: normal. ANA: negative.

Question: What is the diagnosis and recommended therapy?

Diagnosis: Chronic graft-versus-host disease

Discussion: Graft-versus-host disease (GVHD) produces significant morbidity and mortality among patients who have undergone allogeneic bone marrow transplantation (BMT). Acute GVHD usually occurs within 7 to 30 days following BMT and is characterized by fever, rash, hepatitis, and diarrhea. Cutaneous manifestations of acute GVHD include a maculopapular rash, a scarlatiniform rash, and toxic epidermal necrolysis. After the acute phase, cutaneous manifestations evolve from desquamation to hyperpigmentation.

Clinical features of chronic GVHD resemble those of several autoimmune diseases, including scleroderma, systemic lupus erythematosus, and Sjögren's syndrome. Chronic GVHD has a variable onset and may even occur in patients with no known prior episode of acute GVHD. In the early phase of chronic GVHD, the skin lesion resembles lichen planus, primarily involving the buccal mucosa and less frequently the genital mucosa and skin. Direct immunofluorescence reveals immunoglobulin and complement at the dermal-epidermal junction resembling a "lupus band test." In the late phase of chronic GVHD as lichen planus-like lesions fade, the skin assumes a reticulated pigmented and atrophic appearance (poikiloderma).

In some patients with chronic GVHD, the lichen planus-like lesion gives rise to dermal sclerosis resembling that of scleroderma. As in the present case, skin sclerosis begins as a few morphea-like plaques and evolves into extensive cutaneous sclerosis similar to generalized morphea or systemic sclerosis. Unlike systemic sclerosis, in chronic GVHD, acrosclerosis and Raynaud's phenomenon are absent. Many patients with GVHD have autoantibodies including antinuclear, anti-smooth muscle, anti-mitochondrial, and anti-epidermal antibodies, but scleroderma-specific antibodies such as anti-centromere or anti-Scl-70 antibodies usually are not seen.

Another recently described cutaneous manifestation of chronic GVHD is eosinophilic fasciitis. Patients present with the sudden onset of painful swelling of the skin, often accompanied by eosinophilia, that gradually evolves to dermal sclerosis with a *peau d'orange* appearance. Fasciitis may occur as long as 10 years after BMT and may lead to significant disability from joint stiffness and contractures.

Early treatment of chronic GVHD with an alternate-day regimen of cyclosporin A (CyA) and prednisone has led to improved disability-free survival. With the introduction of this form of therapy for chronic GVHD, the incidence of disabling scleroderma-like disease has fallen from 50% to 6%. For patients who do not respond to CyA and prednisone, sclerodermatous manifestations of chronic GVHD may respond to PUVA-therapy, extracorporeal photopheresis, or thalidomide treatment.

The present patient's sclerodermatous skin changes resolved on an alternate-day regimen of CyA and prednisone. Mottled skin pigmentation persisted, but skin thickness returned to normal.

Clinical Pearls

1. Skin thickening without Raynaud's phenomenon or acrosclerosis should suggest a diagnosis of pseudo-scleroderma, one cause of which is chronic GVHD.

2. Although features of autoimmunity such as autoantibodies are frequently present in chronic GVHD, scleroderma-specific autoantibodies such as anti-centromere or anti-Scl-70 antibodies usually are not seen.

3. Eosinophilic fasciitis is a rare, late complication of allogeneic BMT.

4. The incidence of sclerodermatous manifestations of chronic GVHD has declined since the introduction of alternate-day CyA and prednisone immunosuppressive therapy.

REFERENCES

1. Saurat JH. Cutaneous manifestations of graft-versus-host disease. J Dermatol 1981;20:249–256.
2. Rouquette-Gally AM, Boyeldieu D, Prost AC, et al. Autoimmunity after allogeneic bone marrow transplantation. A study of 53 long-term-surviving patients. Transplant 1988;46:238–240.
3. Janin A, Socie G, Devergie A, et al. Fasciitis in chronic graft-versus-host disease. A clinicopathologic study of 14 cases. Ann Intern Med 1994;120:993–998.
4. Siadak M, Sullivan KM. The management of chronic graft-versus-host disease. Blood Rev 1994;8:154–160.

PATIENT 29

A 46-year-old woman with bilateral hip osteoarthritis and cataract

A 46-year-old woman was referred for evaluation and treatment of osteoarthritis. She noted the insidious onset of right hip pain 2 years earlier. Evaluation at that time revealed severe degenerative joint disease, for which she underwent right total hip replacement (THR). One year later she had severe left hip pain after lifting a heavy flowerpot. She was found to have avascular necrosis and degenerative hip disease, and left THR was performed. Subsequently she developed pain in the knees, ankles, hand, wrists, and shoulders.

Her past history was remarkable for long-standing myopia and vitreous degeneration. At age 36, she underwent cataract removal and lens replacement. She received oral prednisone therapy for brief periods after surgery. She was taking steroid eyedrops and a nonsteroidal anti-inflammatory drug.

The family history was significant for early-onset, severe osteoarthritis in her mother, two maternal aunts, and both sisters, one of whom required bilateral THR at age 44.

Physical Examination: Vital signs: normal. General appearance: antalgic gait requiring the use of a walking cane. Skin: normal. HEENT: anterior lens displacement, OD. Neck: normal. Chest: normal. Cardiac: normal. Abdomen: normal. Neurologic: normal. Musculoskeletal: Heberden and Bouchard nodes affecting both hands; crepitus and pain on motion of each first carpometacarpal joints; bilateral genu valgus with crepitus and pain on motion; full, nontender range of motion of both hips status post THR.

Laboratory Findings: CBC: normal. Serum chemistries: normal. Urinalysis: normal. Sedimentation rate: normal. RF: negative. Radiographs of the hips prior to THR: see below.

Question: What is the diagnosis?

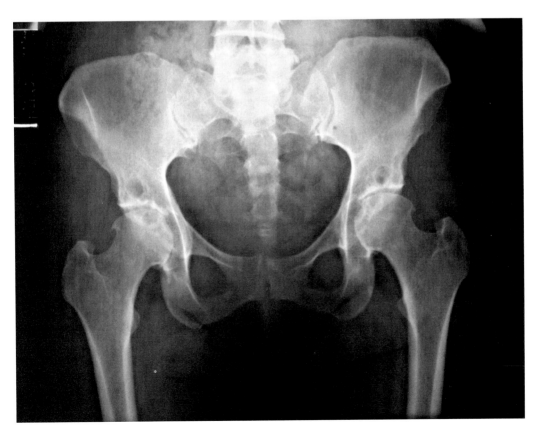

Diagnosis: Stickler syndrome (progressive arthro-ophthalmopathy).

Discussion: Osteoarthritis (OA), the most common joint disease, is characterized by progressive degeneration of cartilage and formation of new bone in subchondral trabeculae and at joint margins (osteophytes). The cardinal clinical feature of OA is pain that is worsened by activity and improved by rest. Other features include gelling, i.e., stiffness after periods of immobility; limitation of motion; and, in extreme cases, functional disability. OA of the hip usually is characterized by insidious onset of pain localized to the groin or medial thigh, followed by a limp. Hip pain is sometimes referred to the knee. In addition to the hips, classic target joints of OA include the interphalangeal and carpometacarpal joints of the hands, the knees and the spine. Other joints whose involvement is less usual include the metacarpal phalangeal joints, the elbows, the shoulders and the ankles. One should consider occupational trauma or metabolic diseases when unusual joints are involved by OA. Joint examination reveals bony enlargement due to new bone formation, e.g., Heberden and Bouchard nodes, tenderness, crepitus, and loss of motion. Radiographic signs of OA are joint space narrowing, subchondral sclerosis, marginal osteophytes, and cyst formation.

OA is a ubiquitous disease. More than 80% of those over age 75 are affected by OA. When OA occurs in a young individual one should consider genetic or metabolic causes. In the present patient, there was disabling OA at a young age and a strong family history of similar joint disease occurring before age 40. Heritable causes of premature OA include metabolic disorders such as hemochromatosis, alkaptonuria, Wilson's disease, and familial chondrocalcinosis. Other genetic causes of premature OA involve defects in type II collagen and have been termed "type II collagenopathies." Type II collagen is found in articular cartilage, the vitreous, and the nucleus pulposus.

Stickler syndrome or hereditary arthro-ophthalmopathy, one of the type II collagenopathies, was first described in 1965. It is a relatively common, yet often undiagnosed, autosomal dominant condition. The incidence of Stickler syndrome has been estimated at 1 in 10,000, making it more common than either Marfan syndrome or osteogenesis imperfecta (1 in 25,000). Failure to diagnose Stickler syndrome may occur because its signs vary widely and only minor features may be present or because physicians often fail to obtain a detailed family history. A diagnosis of Stickler syndrome should be entertained whenever premature OA is diagnosed, particularly if there is a family history of premature OA.

The cardinal features of Stickler syndrome involve the eyes, face, and joints. Ocular manifestations include vitreous degeneration, myopia and cataract as in the present patient, plus retinal detachment. Orofacial features are variable, often recognized in infancy and include midfacial flattening, micrognathia, and the Pierre Robin anomaly (hypognathia, cleft palate, and glossoptosis). Deafness, either sensorineural or conductive, is present in some cases. Premature large joint OA, especially of the hips, as present in this patient and her family is characteristic of Stickler syndrome.

The ocular, orofacial and articular manifestations of Stickler syndrome appear in many cases to result from mutations in the type II procollagen gene (COL2A1). Defects in the same gene may lead to other phenotypic alterations including spondyloepiphyseal dysplasia, hypochondrogenesis, and the Kniest syndrome. Together, these conditions might be considered "type II collagenopathies." It is likely that other forms of familial OA stem from different mutations in the type II procollagen gene or from mutations in genes for other extracellular matrix proteins.

Treatment of OA involves physical modalities such as heat and exercise, nonsteroidal anti-inflammatory drugs and, in severe cases, reconstructive joint surgery. As in the present patient, severe OA of the hip is best managed by THR. Intra-articular corticosteroid therapy may be useful if used judiciously, but oral or parenteral corticosteroids should be avoided. Short courses of oral corticosteroids prescribed for eye disease may have complicated the hip disease by inducing avascular necrosis in the present patient.

Clinical Pearls

1. The classic target joints of OA are the interphalangeal and first carpometacarpal joints of the hands, the hips, the knees, and the spine.

2. Metabolic or other heritable causes should be considered in the patient with premature OA or when nonclassic target joints are affected.

3. Stickler syndrome should be suspected in a young adult with OA of the hip, especially if there is a family history of OA or if there is a history of vitreous degeneration, hearing loss or facial anomalies.

4. In some families, the Stickler syndrome is linked to mutations in the gene for type II procollagen.

REFERENCES

1. Stickler GB, Belau PG, Farrel FJ, et al. Hereditary progressive arthro-ophthalmopathy. Mayo Clin Proc 1965;40:433–455.
2. Pyeritz RE. Heritable disorders of connective tissue. In Schumacher HR Jr, Klippel JH, Koopman WJ (eds). Primer on the Rheumatic Diseases, 10th ed. Atlanta, Arthritis Foundation, 1993, pp 249–255.
3. Rai A, Wordsworth P, Coppock JS, et al. Hereditary arthro-ophthalmopathy (Stickler syndrome): A diagnosis to consider in familial premature osteoarthritis. Br J Rheumatol 1994;33:1175–1180.

PATIENT 30

A 36-year-old woman with a chronic skin rash

A 36-year-old woman presented with an 10-year history of rash affecting the skin of the face, hands, and elbows. She described erythema and scaling of the skin over the knuckles, facial erythema, and scaling, erythematous plaques over the elbows. The facial rash worsened with sun exposure. She had occasional myalgias and arthralgias but no other symptoms to suggest connective tissue disease. She denied muscle weakness. Prior treatment with topical corticosteroids was not beneficial.

Physical Examination: Vital signs: normal. Skin: scaling, erythematous, skin eruptions over the interphalangeal and metacarpophalangeal joints of the hands, the elbows and the medial malleoli; marked periungual telangiectasia with abnormal nailfold capillaries (see Figure). HEENT: facial erythema with suffusion of the lower eyelids. Chest: normal. Cardiac: normal. Abdomen: normal. Neurologic: normal. Musculoskeletal: no synovitis; nontender muscles with normal strength of proximal and distal musculature.

Laboratory Findings: CBC: normal. ESR: 6 mm/hr. Serum chemistries: normal. Skin biopsy: consistent with dermatomyositis. CK: 11 IU/L (normal 14–156). Aldolase: 3.1 IU (1.0–7.0). EMG: normal. MRI of lower extremities: no evidence of inflammatory muscle disease. Muscle biopsy: normal. ANA: 1:80, speckled pattern. Antibodies to ENA, Jo-1, PM-1: negative. PFT: normal. Chest radiograph: normal.

Question: What is the diagnosis?

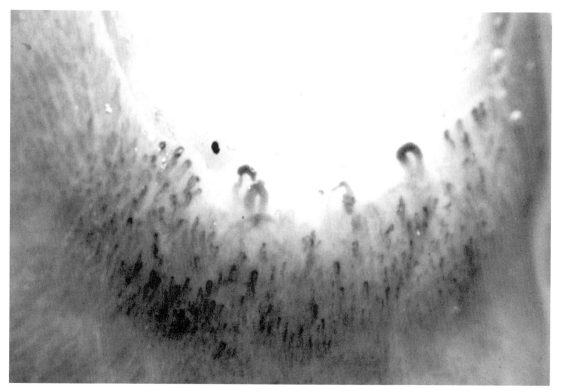

(Provided by HR Maricq)

Diagnosis: Amyopathic dermatomyositis.

Discussion: Dermatomyositis (DM) is an autoimmune disease characterized by an erythematous, photosensitive rash with inflammatory myopathy. Myositis usually results in proximal muscle weakness, myalgia, elevated muscle enzymes (CK and aldolase), abnormal EMG, and inflammation with myonecrosis on muscle biopsy. Autoanti-bodies are usually present, and some patients have myositis-specific antibodies, e.g., anti-Jo-1 and other antisynthetases, anti-signal recognition particle, and anti-Mi-2.

Among the various cutaneous features found in patients with DM is Gottron's sign, erythematous, scaling patches over the dorsal surface of the hands, especially the knuckles, elbows, knees, and medial malleoli. Other cutaneous features of DM include: a dusky purple rash over edematous eyelids (heliotrope rash); a photosensitive rash of the malar and periorbital areas; an erythematous photosensitive rash in the V of the neck (V sign) or over the shoulders and upper back (shawl sign); atrophic skin with areas of hypopigmentation and hyperpigmentation (poikiloderma); scaling and roughening of the skin over the lateral aspects and tips of the fingers (mechanic's hands); ulceration and subcutaneous calcifications (calcinosis cutis) seen more frequently in patients with childhood-onset DM; and periungual telangiectasia.

Cutaneous manifestations of DM usually appear with the onset of myositis but occasionally precede or follow its onset. A rare subset of patients with DM has been described in which typical cutaneous manifestations of DM are present in the absence of clinically apparent muscle disease, i.e., normal strength, muscle enzymes, EMG and muscle biopsy. This subset of DM has been termed "amyopathic dermatomyositis," or dermatomyositis *sine* myositis. Many of such patients develop clinical findings of myositis over time; but others, such as the present patient, do not demonstrate weakness, myalgia, or muscle enzyme elevation even long after (a decade) the onset of cutaneous signs of DM. Patients with amyopathic DM are usually Caucasian females with low-titer, speckled ANA but without myositis-specific autoantibodies.

Magnetic resonance imaging (MRI) has proved to be a sensitive method for localizing inflammation of muscle and may be useful in selecting muscle biopsy sites if signs of inflammation are visible on T2-weighted images. The present patient illustrates that even the MRI may be normal in patients with amyopathic DM. A recent study, however, indicates that these patients do have subtle muscle dysfunction. In a group of amyopathic DM patients, all of whom were Caucasian females with good functional status but moderate degrees of fatigue, there was evidence of abnormal muscle energy metabolism on exercise. Using P-31 magnetic resonance spectroscopy (MRS) to measure oxidative capacity and endurance, amyopathic DM patients were found to have normal MRS at rest and at low work loads but could not sustain work loads as long as normal subjects. The MRS of patients with myopathic DM was abnormal even at rest, and these patients were unable to efficiently generate energy for muscle contraction, even at low levels of exercise.

The cutaneous eruptions of DM are often resistant to therapy. In cases of myopathic DM, corticosteroid therapy may successfully control the myositis without improving the skin eruption. In such cases, as well as in amyopathic cases of DM, therapy with hydroxychloroquine may be beneficial, especially when combined with a sunscreen and with mild topical corticosteroid therapy. The present patient's skin rash improved minimally with such treatment.

Clinical Pearls

1. Cutaneous manifestations of DM may precede, accompany, or follow the onset of muscle disease.

2. Gottron's sign, erythematous scaling patches over the dorsal surface of the hands, especially the knuckles, as well as the elbows, knees, and medial malleoli, is pathognomonic of dermatomyositis (DM).

3. A rare subset of DM in which typical cutaneous signs occur in the absence of clinical or laboratory signs of myositis has been termed "amyopathic DM" or dermatomyositis *sine* myositis.

4. MRI is a sensitive method for localizing sites of myositis for biopsy selection in patients with amyopathic DM.

5. When studied by P-31 magnetic resonance spectroscopy, patients with the amyopathic variant of DM have subtle metabolic evidence of muscle dysfunction unmasked by exercise.

REFERENCES

1. Woo TY, Callen JP, Voorhees JJ, et al. Cutaneous lesions of dermatomyositis are improved with hydroxychloroquine. J Am Acad Dermatol 1984;10:592–600.
2. Fraser DD, Frank JA, Dalakas M, et al. Magnetic resonance imaging in the idiopathic inflammatory myopathies. J Rheumatol 1991;18:1693–1700.
3. Stonecipher MR, Jorizzo JL, White WL, et al. Cutaneous changes of dermatomyositis in patients with normal muscle enzymes: dermatomyositis sine myositis? J Am Acad Dermatol 1993;28:951–956.
4. Park JH, Olsen NJ, King L Jr, et al. Use of magnetic resonance imaging and P-31 magnetic resonance spectroscopy to detect and quantify muscle dysfunction in the amyopathic and myopathic variants of dermatomyositis. Arthritis Rheum 1995;38:68–77.

PATIENT 31

A 72-year-old man with arthritis and dyspnea

A 72-year-old man presented with a chief complaint of dyspnea. He had a 4-year history of dyspnea that had worsened significantly during the preceding 6 months. He had a 100-pack per year smoking history and was hospitalized for bronchitis 6 months earlier. He denied wheezing, cough, sputum production, fever, or night sweats. Past history revealed coronary artery angioplasty 7 years earlier and idiopathic nephrotic syndrome. A rectal biopsy for amyloidosis was negative.

The patient had a 24-year history of seropositive, nodular rheumatoid arthritis (RA). Past treatment included intramuscular and oral gold, d-penicillamine, and nonsteroidal anti-inflammatory drugs. At the time of evaluation he was taking aspirin and low-dose prednisone for RA.

Physical Examination: Vital signs: temperature 97.8°; pulse 82; respirations 18; blood pressure 140/80. Skin: subcutaneous nodules over each olecranon process. Lymph nodes: normal. HEENT: normal. Neck: no jugular venous distention. Back: no presacral edema. Chest: end-inspiratory "velcro" rales in the bases. Cardiac: normal. Abdomen: normal. Neurologic: normal. Musculoskeletal: ulnar deviation with swan-neck deformities in both hands; limited abduction and rotation of both shoulders; fibular deviation and metatarsal-phalangeal subluxation affecting both feet; no erythema, warmth, or tenderness. Extremities: clubbing of fingers; bilateral 2+ pretibial edema.

Laboratory Findings: CBC: normal. ESR: 81 mm/hr. Urinalysis: 300 mg/dL protein. BUN 24 mg/dL, albumin 2.5 g/dL, total protein 6.6 g/dL. Rheumatoid factor 1:80. Chest radiograph: see Figure. PFT: FVC 2.79 L (69% of predicted); FEV_1 1.67 L (63% of predicted); FEV_1/FVC 90% of predicted; FEF_{25-75} 36% of predicted; DLCO 16% of predicted; O_2 saturation of 93% at rest and 84% after walking 100 feet.

Question: What is the diagnosis?

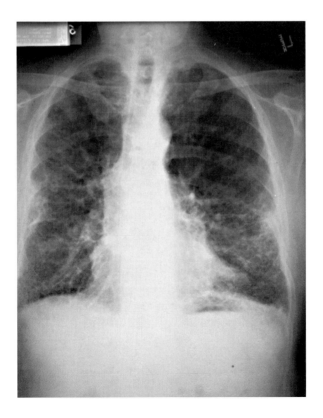

Diagnosis: Rheumatoid interstitial lung disease.

Discussion: Pulmonary manifestations of RA are protean. Occasionally pulmonary features precede the onset of joint disease. The frequency and severity of pulmonary complications are higher among men with RA, particularly the elderly, than among women with RA. The most common pulmonary complications of RA include rheumatoid nodules, pleurisy with effusion, and diffuse pulmonary fibrosis (interstitial lung disease). Less common respiratory problems include upper airway obstruction from cricoarytenoid arthritis, small airways obstruction, Caplan's syndrome and obliterative bronchiolitis.

Caplan's syndrome was described in 1953, and refers to the radiologic appearance of nodular fibrosis in coalminers with coexistent RA. Unlike the fibrosis of simple pneumoconiosis, in Caplan's syndrome the histology shows features of a typical rheumatoid nodule with endarteritis and an enhancing ring of coal dust. Caplan's syndrome is relatively rare in North America but common in Western Europe. Patients are usually asymptomatic, unless lesions cavitate and rupture, producing black sputum and hemoptysis. Breathlessness is unusual.

Pulmonary parenchymal rheumatoid nodules are usually multiple, measuring 1–2 cm in diameter. They are frequently subpleural and may rupture to produce a pneumothorax or pleural effusion. RA patients with pulmonary nodules are often asymptomatic. Rarely, pulmonary nodules cavitate and become colonized by Mycobacterium and Aspergillus.

Pleural effusion is the most common clinical manifestation of rheumatoid lung disease, occurring in up to 10% of cases. Pleural effusions are exudative and characteristically have a low glucose concentration (<30 mg/dL), a low pH (usually 7.00), an LDH > 1000 IU/L, and demonstrate features of immune complex formation and complement consumption. A characteristic cytologic picture of orange-red granular material, large, elongated cells, and giant multinucleated cells. Rheumatoid pleural effusions are often asymptomatic and usually resolve spontaneously over several months.

Although there has been some controversy, it is now evident that the incidence of interstitial lung disease is higher in RA patients than in normal controls. As illustrated by the present patient, rheumatoid interstitial lung disease is predominantly seen in males (4:1) who are seropositive and who have other extra-articular complications, such as rheumatoid nodules. Cigarette smoking has been implicated in the development and severity of rheumatoid interstitial lung disease. Most patients have nonproductive cough and dyspnea on exertion. Clubbing and bibasilar dry crackles may be present. The chest radiograph shows bilateral symmetric reticulonodular markings. Spirometry reveals a restrictive pattern with a decrease in lung volumes and an increase in the FEV/FVC ratio. As in the present patient, a mixed restrictive and obstructive pattern may be seen, especially in the patient with a history of cigarette use. Oxygen transfer is usually impaired, and oxygen saturation will worsen with exercise. In the present patient, progressive pulmonary fibrosis leading to obliteration of the pulmonary microvasculature was the cause of oxygen desaturation.

Although usually a spontaneously occurring process, interstitial lung disease may sometimes be a complication of drug therapy for RA. Gold, d-penicillamine, sulfasalazine, alkylating agents and methotrexate may each produce life-threatening pulmonary disease. The presence of pre-existing lung disease is now regarded as a risk factor for the development of methotrexate pneumonitis. Discontinuation of the implicated drug and treatment with high-dose corticosteroids may be life-saving in such situations.

Treatment of non-drug-induced rheumatoid interstitial lung disease is more problematic and empiric. High-dose oral corticosteroid therapy is beneficial for some patients. The addition of azathioprine or cyclophosphamide may provide further control and may be steroid-sparing. Side-effects of such therapy are seen in up to 30% of cases and include neutropenia, thrombocytopenia, infection, and hemorrhagic cystitis. The worst outcome occurs in patients with a slowly progressive form of the disease who have established fibrosis at the time of initiating therapy and who have granulocytic bronchoalveolar lavage fluid. Bronchoalveolar lavage often yields an excess of lymphocytes, neutrophils, or eosinophils. A lymphocytic pneumonitis is believed to indicate a favorable response to corticosteroid therapy, whereas neutrophil or eosinophil excess is associated with a poor prognosis.

The present patient was thought to have irreversible pulmonary fibrosis and probable pulmonary hypertension. He showed some improvement in dyspnea with an increase in dosage of his corticosteroid therapy and when given supplemental oxygen with exercise.

Clinical Pearls

1. Pulmonary complications of RA are associated with rheumatoid factor positivity, nodules, and male gender and, in some cases, may precede the onset of arthritis.

2. The characteristic pleural fluid typical of rheumatoid pleurisy is a low glucose concentration (<30 mg/dL), a pH of 7.00, and an LDH > 1000 IU/L.

3. Rheumatoid interstitial lung disease is the most likely diagnosis in an RA patient with clubbing and bibasilar crackles.

4. Although rheumatoid interstitial lung disease is usually spontaneous, antirheumatic drugs can produce a hypersensitivity pneumonitis.

5. Pre-existing lung disease with interstitial infiltrates on chest radiography predisposes patients with RA to methotrexate pneumonitis.

REFERENCES

1. Nosanchuk JS, Naylor B. A unique cytologic picture in pleural fluid from patients with rheumatoid arthritis. Am J Clin Path 1968;50:330–335.
2. Kelly CA. Rheumatoid arthritis: classical rheumatoid lung disease. In Kelly CA (ed). Lung Disease in Rheumatic Disorders. Balliere's Clinical Rheumatology. Philadelphia, Balliere Tindall, 1993, pp 1–16.
3. Case records of the Massachusetts General Hospital. Weekly clinicopathological exercises. Case 44–1994. N Engl J Med 1994;331:1642–1647.
4. Golden MR, Katz RS, Balk RA, et al. The relationship of preexisting lung disease to the development of methotrexate pneumonitis in patients with rheumatoid arthritis. J Rheumatol 1995;22:1043–1047.

PATIENT 32

A 46-year-old woman with unilateral hand pain

A 46-year-old right-handed female Corrections Officer presented with a several month history of pain in her dominant hand. She recalled no history of trauma, but her job included manual labor. The pain involved the dorsal and ventral aspects of the wrist and it was exacerbated by writing. She denied swelling, erythema, or warmth of the wrist or hand joints. Her past medical history was remarkable for cervical disc disease for which she had a cervical laminectomy several years prior to the onset of the wrist pain.

Physical Examination: Vital signs: normal. General: normal. Neurologic examination: negative Tinel sign over the median nerve and negative Phalen sign; sensation and motor strength normal; DTR's 2 + bilaterally. Musculoskeletal: mild tenderness over the right wrist with pain on extension and flexion; no swelling, warmth or erythema.

Laboratory Findings: CBC, chemistries, and ESR: normal. EMG/NCV: normal. MRI of cervical spine: central disc bulge at C3-C4 and s/p fusion at C5-C6. Radiograph of the wrist: see Figure.

Question: What is the diagnosis?

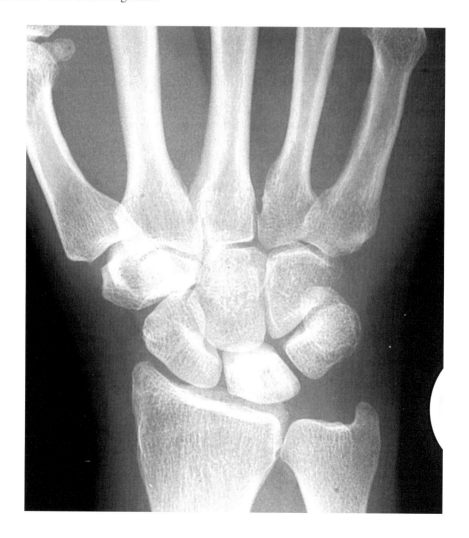

Diagnosis: Kienböck disease (osteonecrosis of the lunate)

Discussion: Osteonecrosis of the carpal lunate is known as Kienböck disease. Although the cause is unknown, Kienböck disease has a predilection for the right hand in individuals engaged in manual labor, as in the present patient. Bilateral involvement has been described less frequently. Because it usually is unilateral and involves the dominant hand, Kienböck disease is believed to arise from trauma. Indeed, a history of trauma is often but not always elicited. In some cases the trauma may have been trivial or isolated, whereas in other cases there is a history of repetitive trauma related to occupational or recreational usage. Other sites of osteonecrosis believed to be associated with trauma are the metatarsal head (Freiberg disease), the capitulum of the humerus (Panner disease), and the phalanges of the hand (Thiemann disease).

Progressive pain, swelling and disability occur often. Other causes of hand pain such as cervical radiculopathy, carpal tunnel syndrome, reflex sympathetic dystrophy syndrome (RSDS), or arthritis usually can be differentiated from the pain of Kienböck disease. In the present patient there was no evidence of RSDS or compression neuropathy, nor was there serologic or radiographic evidence of arthritis. Although the patient had cervical disc disease, the normal neurologic examination and EMG/NCV militate against cervical radiculopathy as a cause of the wrist pain.

Kienböck disease is diagnosed by distinctive changes seen on radiography. As in the present patient, increased density of the lunate relative to the other carpal bones is evident (see Figure). Tomography may reveal a linear or compression fracture prior to the sclerotic stage. In an early stage, bone scintigraphy and MR imaging are sensitive and specific, respectively. Eventually, the lunate may collapse and fragment. Complications include disruption of the normal carpal architecture, scapulolunate separation, ulnar deviation of the triquetrum, and secondary degenerative arthritis of the radiocarpal and midcarpal joints. Tendons may be eroded and may rupture secondary to a distorted and collapsed lunate.

The pathogenesis of Kienböck disease involves both fracture and osteonecrosis. Two features predisposing the lunate to injury and subsequent osteonecrosis have been proposed: (1) a fixed position in the wrist resulting in mechanical forces that exceed those on the other carpal bones; and (2) a vulnerable blood supply arising from vessels entering on the dorsal and volar sides and anastomosing within it. Up to 26% of individuals may lack either a dorsal or volar arterial supply. It is unclear whether a short ulna predisposes to Kienböck disease by increasing the mechanical forces on the lunate, but a short ulna (ulna minus variant) is seen in as many as 75% of cases.

Various forms of treatment have been advocated, including ulnar lengthening, radial shortening, and lunate replacement. Secondary degenerative changes had not yet occurred in the present patient, and her symptoms improved with splinting and nonsteroidal anti-inflammatory drugs.

Clinical Pearls

1. Kienböck disease refers to osteonecrosis of the carpal lunate and should be considered in a patient who complains of pain in the dominant hand, especially if there is a history of trauma.

2. In the early stage of Kienböck disease, the radiographs reveal increased density of the lunate without alteration of the shape of the bone; later, there is collapse of the sclerotic lunate bone.

3. Other trauma-induced sites of osteonecrosis include the metatarsal head (Freiberg infraction), the capitulum of the humerus (Panner disease), and the phalanges of the hands (Thiemann disease).

REFERENCES

1. Reiners WR, Conway WF, Totty WG, et al. Carpal avascular necrosis: MR imaging. Radiology 1986;160:689–693.
2. Resnick D. Osteochondroses. In Resnick D, Niwayama G (eds). Diagnosis of Bone and Joint Disorders, 2d ed. Philadelphia, WB Saunders, 1988, pp 3288–3334.
3. Williams CS, Gelberman RH. Vascularity of the lunate. Anatomic studies and implications for the development of osteonecrosis. Hand Clin. 1993;9:391–398.

PATIENT 33

A 7-year-old girl with weakness, rash, and fever

A 7-year-old girl fell 2 days before presentation and struck her elbow. The following morning she awoke with pain, swelling, and warmth at the site of the injury. She had a 2-year history of rash involving the eyelids, elbows, knuckles, and knees. She was also noted to have malaise and fatigue and was unable to keep up with the activities of other children. Specifically, she found it difficult to walk upstairs or arise from a sitting position.

Physical Examination: Temperature 103.3°, pulse 140, respirations 20, blood pressure 103/61. General appearance: alert, cooperative child guarding the left elbow. Skin: erythema and hyperpigmentation of the skin over both upper eyelids and malar area; erythematous papules over the extensor surface of the knees and knuckles of both hands; subcutaneous nodules present in the area of each olecranon with a cutaneous ulceration over the left olecranon exuding purulent fluid containing a chalky white material. HEENT: normal. Chest: clear. Cardiac: normal. Abdomen: normal. Neurologic: normal. Musculoskeletal: proximal muscle strength 3/5 and distal muscle strength 5/5; joints normal except for left elbow, which was warm, erythematous, and tender to touch; elbow pronation and supination normal, but flexion and extension markedly reduced due to pain.

Laboratory Findings: Hct 36.6%; WBC 20,600/μL with 67% neutrophils, 11% bands, 3% monocytes, 18% lymphocytes, and 1% eosinophils; platelets 201,000/μL; ESR 20 mm/hr; serum electrolytes normal; CPK 147 IU/L (20–270); aldolase 15.7 IU/L (1.0–7.0). Blood culture: no growth. Left elbow exudate: few leukocytes, gram-positive cocci in pairs with heavy growth of *Staphylococcus aureus*. Radiographs of left elbow: see Figure.

Question: How would you treat the acute complication of this child's chronic condition?

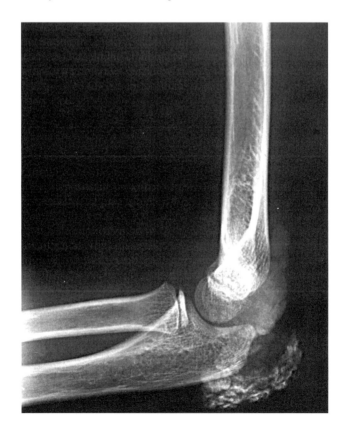

Diagnosis: Juvenile dermatomyositis with calcinosis and acute staphylococcal cellulitis.

Discussion: Dermatomyositis with onset in childhood (juvenile dermatomyositis) is a chronic idiopathic inflammatory myositis associated with characteristic skin lesions. The etiology is unknown, but early lesions of the skin and muscle are characterized by a vasculopathy. Immunohistochemical stains reveal deposition of the complement membrane attack complex within the microvasculature of muscle. The diagnosis of juvenile dermatomyositis is based on the following criteria: (1) symmetric proximal muscle weakness; (2) characteristic cutaneous changes consisting of periorbital edema with a heliotrope discoloration of the eyelids, and a scaly rash over the extensor aspect of the MCP, interphalangeal, elbow and knee joints (Gottron's papules); (3) elevation of serum levels of one or more muscle enzymes (creatine kinase, aldolase, lactic dehydrogenase, aspartate aminotransferase); (4) inflammatory myopathic changes on electromyogram; (5) muscle biopsy showing histologic evidence of necrosis and inflammation. The differential diagnosis includes postviral myositis, primary myopathies, and inflammatory myositis accompanying another connective tissue disease.

Calcinosis occurs in up to 75% of children with juvenile dermatomyositis. The clinical presentation of calcinosis is variable and unpredictable, ranging from 4 months to over 10 years after onset of disease. Dystrophic calcification occurs as superficial plaques or nodules, deep tumorous deposits in proximal muscles (calcinosis circumscripta), or deposition within intermuscular fascial planes (calcinosis universalis), each of which may interfere with joint or muscle function. Subcutaneous calcification is often associated with ulceration of overlying skin and is observed more frequently than calcification in intermuscular fascial planes. Subcutaneous calcinosis is seen most commonly around the knees and elbows (see Figure) and in the fingers.

In juvenile dermatomyositis ulceration of the skin may occur secondary to cutaneous vasculitis or secondary to the extrusion of calcific material from underlying nodules. In the latter case, surgical excision of calcigerous material is sometimes required. Such cases may be complicated by secondary infection as in the present case, or by an inflammatory response to hydroxyapatite crystals. Numerous reports of regression of calcinosis in children treated with various therapies have been published. Most recently there have been reports of regression of calcinosis in two scleroderma patients treated with the calcium channel blocker, diltiazem. Spontaneous resolution of calcinosis in juvenile dermatomyositis has been observed, indicating the need for caution in interpretation of any such reports claiming efficacy of drug therapy.

In the present patient, the presence of the characteristic rash, proximal muscle weakness, and elevated serum aldolase confirmed the diagnosis of juvenile dermatomyositis. Calcific material drained spontaneously from the lesion overlying the elbow. Radiographs revealed soft tissue calcification and soft tissue swelling posterior to the elbow joint. Secondary cellulitis caused by *Staphylococcus aureus* responded to antibiotic therapy and wound care. The skin lesion healed and the child regained full range of motion of the elbow. Weakness and enzyme elevation responded to corticosteroid therapy, but the rash persisted.

Clinical Pearls

1. Juvenile dermatomyositis is frequently complicated by dystrophic calcifications.

2. Calcinosis may occur as superficial nodules, deep tumorous deposits in proximal muscles (calcinosis circumscripta), or deposition within intermuscular fascial planes (calcinosis universalis).

3. Ulceration of the skin overlying subcutaneous calcinosis can be complicated by infection requiring antibiotic therapy and, at times, surgical excision of calcigerous material.

4. A high rate of spontaneous regression complicates evaluation of the efficacy of proposed anticalcinotic therapy.

REFERENCES
1. Sewell JR, Liyanage B, Ansell BM. Calcinosis in juvenile dermatomyositis. Skeletal Radiol 1978;3:137–143.
2. Kissel JT, Mendell JR, Rammohan KW. Microvascular deposition of complement membrane attack complex in dermatomyositis. N Engl J Med 1986;314:329–334.
3. Juvenile Dermatomyositis. In Cassidy JT, Petty RE (eds). Textbook of Pediatric Rheumatology, 3d ed. Philadelphia, WB Saunders, 1995, pp 323–364.
4. Dolan AL, Kassimos D, Gibson T, et al. Diltiazem induces remission of calcinosis in scleroderma. Br J Rheumatol 1995;34:576–578.

PATIENT 34

A 14-year-old girl with swelling of the arms and legs

A 14-year-old girl presented with a 3-month history of swelling of the arms and legs. Her illness began as morning stiffness in the upper arms followed by pitting edema of the arms and legs. A urinalysis revealed only 1⁺ proteinuria, and the blood pressure was normal. A CBC revealed 12.5% eosinophils, and she was referred for further evaluation. Additional history revealed a complaint of tight skin of the arms and hands that interfered with her piano lessons. There was no history of Raynaud's phenomenon, nor was there dyspnea or dysphagia. She described nocturnal paresthesias of the fingers.

Physical Examination: Temperature 97.9°; pulse 112; respirations 20; blood pressure 110/70. Skin: taut skin over the upper (forearms > arms) and lower (legs > thighs) extremities without sclerodactyly, telangiectasia, or truncal scleroderma. HEENT: normal. Chest: normal. Cardiac: normal. Abdomen: normal. Neurologic: normal. Musculoskeletal: mildly limited flexion and extension of the wrists and MCP joints. Extremities: mild, nonpitting edema of the legs.

Laboratory Findings: WBC 5900/µL with 50% neutrophils, 30% lymphocytes, 10% monocytes, and 10% eosinophils; Hct 33.5%; platelets 222,000/µL; electrolytes normal; Cr 0.8 mg/dL; urinalysis normal; liver function tests normal; CPK normal; aldolase 13.4 IU/L (0–7 IU/L); ANA, RF and Scl-70 antibody negative; serum complements normal. Nailfold capillary microscopy: normal. MRI of legs: see below.

Question: What is the cause of this child's swelling and eosinophilia?

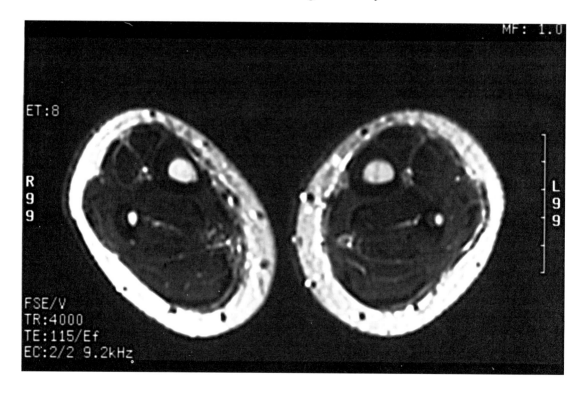

Diagnosis: Childhood-onset eosinophilic fasciitis.

Discussion: Eosinophilic fasciitis was first described as a distinct clinical entity by Shulman in 1974, and consists of diffuse fasciitis, peripheral blood eosinophilia and hypergammaglobulinemia. The skin of the upper and/or lower extremities is indurated, painful, and edematous. Unlike scleroderma, in eosinophilic fasciitis patients usually do not have Raynaud's phenomenon, sclerodactyly or facial skin sclerosis, gastrointestinal or cardiopulmonary involvement, nor do they exhibit the characteristic nailfold capillary abnormalities seen in scleroderma. Although the ANA may be positive in eosinophilic fasciitis, scleroderma-specific autoantibodies (anti-centromere and anti-Scl-70 antibodies) are absent. The etiology of eosinophilic fasciitis is unknown. Its onset has been associated with strenuous physical exertion in many cases and exposure to the solvent trichlorethylene in two reported cases.

Eosinophilic fasciitis rarely occurs in childhood. Childhood onset has been distinguished from adult onset by the preponderance of females, increased involvement of muscle with eosinophilic infiltrates, and lack of hematologic complications such as thrombocytopenia or aplastic anemia. In both children and adults with eosinophilic fasciitis, there is a lack of visceral organ involvement and a variable response to steroid therapy.

The present patient was diagnosed by the clinical findings of symmetric extremity swelling and induration; the absence of scleroderma features such as Raynaud's phenomenon, sclerodactyly or capillary abnormalities; and the blood eosinophilia. The mildly elevated serum aldolase with a normal CK level is also characteristic of diffuse fasciitis. Other indurative skin conditions in children include morphea, linear scleroderma, scleredema, and rare genetic conditions such as phenylketonuria, Werner syndrome, and Winchester syndrome.

The gold-standard diagnostic test for eosinophilic fasciitis has been the full-thickness skin biopsy that includes skin, fascia, and underlying muscle. Findings in adult- and childhood-onset eosinophilic fasciitis include perivascular mononuclear cell infiltrates in the lower dermis and subcutis, thickened fascia with inflammatory cell infiltrates composed of lymphocytes, plasma cells, histocytes, and usually eosinophils. Magnetic resonance imaging (MRI) has been shown to be a useful noninvasive tool for diagnosing eosinophilic fasciitis. T2-weighted images demonstrate thickening and hyperintensity of the fascia. In the present case there was increased signal intensity on T2-weighted images in the deep transverse fascia posterior to the tibialis posterior muscles in the upper calves (see Figure). Such changes have been shown to resolve with steroid therapy.

Approximately one-third of children with eosinophilic fasciitis experience complete resolution, while the remainder are left with residual cutaneous fibrosis.

The present child was treated with prednisone (1 mg/kg/d), which was accompanied by normalization of the CBC and prompt improvement in the swelling of the extremities. The prednisone was tapered and discontinued with the only residual abnormality being mild flexion contractures of the second and third MCP joints due to cutaneous fibrosis.

Clinical Pearls

1. Eosinophilic fasciitis is characterized by symmetric induration, pain and edema of the upper and/or lower extremities in association with blood eosinophilia and hypergammaglobulinemia.

2. Eosinophilic fasciitis is distinguished from scleroderma by the absence of visceral involvement, Raynaud's phenomenon, capillary abnormalities, sclerodactyly or facial involvement, and by the absence of scleroderma-specific antibodies.

3. Eosinophilic fasciitis occurs rarely in children and must be distinguished from scleroderma, morphea, scleredema, phenylketonuria, and other rare genetic diseases.

4. Magnetic resonance imaging (MRI) is a noninvasive method that may aid in diagnosing eosinophilic fasciitis, either by selecting a site for biopsy or by confirming the clinical impression of fasciitis, and may prove useful in monitoring the response to treatment.

REFERENCES

1. Grisanti MW, Moore TL, Osborn TG, Haber PL. Eosinophilic fasciitis in children. Semin Arthritis Rheum 1989;19:151–157.
2. Falanga V. Fibrosing conditions in childhood. Adv Dermatol 1991;6:145–158.
3. Farrington ML, Haas JE, Nazar-Stewart V, Mellins ED. Eosinophilic fasciitis in children frequently progresses to scleroderma-like cutaneous fibrosis. J Rheumatol 1993;20:128–132.
4. al-Shaikh A, Freeman C, Avruch L, McKendry RJ. Use of magnetic resonance imaging in diagnosing eosinophilic fasciitis. Report of two cases. Arthritis Rheum 1994;37:1602–1608.

PATIENT 35

A 59-year-old woman with scleroderma and progressive dyspnea

A 59-year-old woman with scleroderma was referred because of progressive dyspnea. She had a 2 year history of skin tightness, Raynaud's phenomenon, and dyspepsia and was found to have scleroderma with anti-Scl-70 antibodies. She complained of dyspnea on exertion (1 flight) with a nonproductive cough, and her pulmonary function deteriorated despite treatment with d-penicillamine and nifedipine.

Physical Examination: Temperature 98.5°; pulse 96; respirations 24; blood pressure 134/80. Skin: sclerodactyly and scleroderma affecting the upper extremities, face, and neck. HEENT: normal. Neck: no jugular venous distension. Back: normal. Chest: diminished breath sounds with bibasilar rales. Cardiac: normal. Abdomen: normal. Neurologic: normal. Musculoskeletal: flexion contractures of fingers, wrists and elbows due to skin sclerosis.

Laboratory Findings: WBC 9,600/μL; Hct 41.3%; platelet count 305,000/μL. BUN 10 mg/dL; urinalysis normal. Westergren ESR 37 mm/hr. ANA positive, 1:640 with speckled pattern; Scl-70 antibody positive; RNP, Smith, ENA negative. Chest radiograph: bibasilar fibrotic changes with normal cardiac silhouette. Pulmonary function tests: FVC 1.38L (44% predicted); FEV_1, 0.94L (41% predicted); FEV_1/FVC 92%; DL_{co} 5.6 mL/min/mmHg (26% predicted). Bronchoalveolar lavage: 68 × 10⁶ cells with 72% alveolar macrophages, 12% lymphocytes and 16% neutrophils. High-resolution computed tomography (HRCT) of chest: see Figure.

Question: What is the cause of this patient's progressive dyspnea?

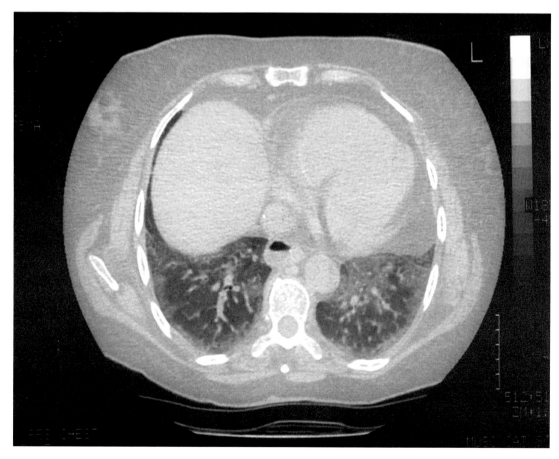

Diagnosis: Scleroderma lung disease with active alveolitis.

Discussion: Scleroderma frequently involves the lungs, and lung disease is a major cause of morbidity and mortality among scleroderma patients. Pulmonary manifestations are protean and include interstitial fibrosis, pulmonary hypertension, aspiration pneumonia, carcinoma of the lung, pleurisy, pneumothorax, and silicosis. Rare patients may present with interstitial lung disease before the onset of skin involvement (systemic sclerosis *sine* scleroderma). Such patients can be distinguished from patients with idiopathic pulmonary fibrosis (IPF) by the presence of Raynaud's phenomenon, abnormal nailfold capillaries, and esophageal dysmotility.

Interstitial lung disease associated with scleroderma has surpassed renovascular hypertension as a cause of death. Risk factors for scleroderma lung fibrosis include diffuse cutaneous sclerosis and the presence of anti-Scl-70 antibodies. Patients with scleroderma lung disease complain of dyspnea and a nonproductive cough. On examination, fine bibasilar rales are heard. Chest radiographs may show bibasilar fibrosis, and PFTs show a restrictive pattern. Such traditional tests of lung disease, however, have not been shown to be predictive of pulmonary outcome.

Two newer techniques that have shown promise in predicting outcome are bronchoalveolar lavage (BAL) and high-resolution computed tomography (HRCT) of the chest. Scleroderma patients whose BAL yields an increased total number of cells with a neutrophilic alveolitis are at high risk for deteriorating pulmonary function. In such cases HRCT often demonstrates reticular markings and a ground-glass opacification, particularly in the posterobasilar segments, as seen in the present case (see Figure). Other HRCT findings in scleroderma include hilar and mediastinal lymphadenopathy, irregular pleural margins, subpleural cysts and bronchiectasis.

The present patient had findings on BAL and HRCT of active alveolitis while being treated with d-penicillamine (DPA). DPA has not been shown to alter the course of scleroderma lung disease. Three uncontrolled studies suggest, however, that cyclophosphamide treatment may improve pulmonary function (FVC) in scleroderma patients with active interstitial lung disease. The present patient was treated with daily oral cyclophosphamide (125 mg/d). After 6 months, her dyspnea was improved and the FVC was 1.65L (53% predicted).

Clinical Pearls

1. Interstitial lung disease is now the leading cause of death among scleroderma patients.

2. Diffuse cutaneous systemic sclerosis and the presence of anti-Scl-70 antibodies are risk factors for scleroderma interstitial lung disease.

3. Rare patients may present with lung disease before the onset of skin sclerosis (systemic sclerosis *sine* scleroderma).

4. Deterioration in lung function may be predicted by a neutrophilic alveolitis on BAL.

5. The HRCT finding of ground-glass opacification has been associated with a neutrophilic alveolitis by BAL and an active inflammatory interstitial lesion by open-lung biopsy.

REFERENCES

1. Manuossakis MN, Constantopoulos SH, Gharavi AE, Moutsopoulos HM. Pulmonary involvement in systemic sclerosis. Association with anti-Scl-70 antibody and digital pitting. Chest 1987;92:509–513.
2. Lomeo RM, Cornella RJ, Schabel SI, Silver RM. Progressive systemic sclerosis *sine* scleroderma presenting as pulmonary interstitial fibrosis. Am J Med 1989;87:525–527.
3. Silver RM, Miller KS, Kinsella MB, Smith EA, Schabel SI. Evaluation and management of scleroderma lung disease using bronchoalveolar lavage. Am J Med 1990;88:470–475.
4. Altman RD, Medsger TA Jr, Block DA, Michel BA. Predictors of survival in systemic sclerosis (scleroderma). Arthritis Rheum 1991;34:403–413.
5. Warrick JH, Bhalla M, Schabel SI, Silver RM. High resolution computed tomography in early scleroderma lung disease. J Rheumatol 1991;18:1520–1528.
6. Silver RM, Warrick JH, Kinsella MB, Staudt LS, Baumann MH, Strange C. Cyclosphosphamide and low-dose prednisone therapy in patients with systemic sclerosis (scleroderma) with interstitial lung disease. J Rheumatol 1993;20:838–844.

PATIENT 36

An 8-year-old boy with fever, rash, and arthritis

An 8-year-old boy was well until he developed an erythematous rash beginning on his back, accompanied by painful swelling of both ankles. The ankle arthritis resolved after several days, but he developed arthritis of the right wrist and a sustained fever up to 103°. The rash spread rapidly over the trunk, arms and thighs; individual lesions showed rapid outward expansion of serpiginous, annular, and polycyclic papules for 4 to 6 hours. A younger sibling had streptococcal pharyngitis and scarlet fever 6 weeks earlier. His maternal grandmother had a history of JRA. The patient was allergic to penicillin.

Physical Examination: Temperature 99.6°; heart rate 90, regular; respiratory rate 20; blood pressure 90/58. Skin: annular urticarial lesions with central clearing on the back, chest, thighs and arms (see Figure). Nodes: shotty cervical adenopathy. HEENT: mild pharyngeal injection. Chest: clear. Cardiovascular: regular rate and rhythm with Grade I/VI systolic murmur. Abdomen: normal. Neurologic: normal. Musculoskeletal: normal.

Laboratory Findings: Hct 35.3%; WBC 12,700/µL with 74% neutrophils, 15% lymphocytes, 2% monocytes, 2% eosinophils, 5% reactive lymphocytes and 2% bands; platelets 425,000/µL; Westergren ESR 82 mm/hr; ANA negative; RF negative; throat culture negative for beta hemolytic streptococci; streptozyme positive, 1:400; ASO titer 480 Todd units; CRP 8.9 (0.0–0.8); ECG normal; echocardiogram normal.

Question: What is the rash and the diagnosis?

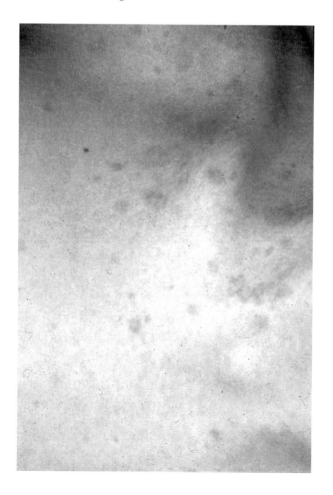

Diagnosis: Erythema marginatum and acute rheumatic fever.

Discussion: Erythema marginatum is an uncommon manifestation of acute rheumatic fever (ARF), occurring in fewer than 10% of children with this disorder. Its presence indicates a higher risk for the development of carditis. Erythema marginatum is one of five major manifestations of ARF, together with carditis, polyarthritis, chorea, and subcutaneous nodules. The revised modified Jones criteria for the diagnosis of ARF requires the presence of two major criteria, or one major and two minor criteria, supported by evidence of a preceding streptococcal infection (increased ASO titer, positive pharyngeal culture, recent scarlet fever). The minor criteria are fever, arthralgia, previous rheumatic carditis, prolonged PR interval, and an increased ESR or C-reactive protein.

Two childhood rheumatic diseases that can mimic ARF are systemic-onset juvenile arthritis (Still's disease) and systemic lupus erythematosus (SLE). Still's disease may present with fever, arthritis, and evanescent rash. Unlike ARF, the fever of Still's disease usually has a quotidian pattern and the maculopapular rash of Still's disease is most pronounced at the height of the fever. In each condition the rash may be evanescent and show central pallor. In SLE, the classic rash is malar erythema or a discoid lesion, and the ANA is nearly always positive. Erythema marginatum is readily distinguishable from other childhood diseases characterized by

Henoch-Schönlein purpura, and erythema infectiosum.

Arthritis is the most common major manifestation of ARF. Joint pain is often severe and out of proportion to objective signs of arthritis. Classically, it is polyarticular and migratory, with a predilection for large lower extremity joints. Arthritis in any one joint resolves within several weeks, unlike juvenile chronic arthritis which persists for 6 weeks or longer. The arthralgia and arthritis of ARF respond dramatically to salicylates.

In the present case, this boy had an acute onset of evanescent rash, high fever, and arthritis. A diagnosis of acute rheumatic fever was made on the basis of polyarthritis and erythema marginatum with fever, an elevated ESR, and CRP, plus evidence of a preceding streptococcal infection. Although rare, there has been a resurgence of acute rheumatic fever in developed countries. His fever and arthritis resolved within days of beginning aspirin, 650 mg tid (70 mg/kg/d). Aspirin was discontinued because of gastrointestinal tract upset several weeks later, and high fever and rash returned. These symptoms subsided with the administration of tolmetin (30 mg/kg/d). The rash resolved gradually, and the patient was asymptomatic and the ESR was 17 mm/hr when seen 6 weeks later. In view of the history of allergy to penicillin, he was placed on sulfadiazine, 500 mg daily, as prophylaxis of rheumatic heart disease.

earls

of acute rheumatic fever, erythema marthan 10% of patients with this condition.

inless, usually flat, spreading rash that

early stage of ARF and is often associ-

eumatic fever in the intermountain area of the United States.

natic fever: early diagnosis by skin biopsy. J Am Acad Dermatol

histopathologic manifestation. J Am Acad Dermatol 1989;

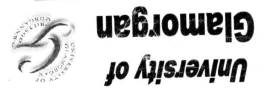

PATIENT 37

A 63-year-old woman with polyarthralgias and hoarseness

A 63-year-old woman with essential hypertension was well until her dose of hydralazine was increased from 100 mg to 200 mg daily. For the previous 7 years she had taken hydralazine, 100 mg daily, without untoward effects. Within 1 month of the change in dose, symmetric polyarthralgias involving wrists, elbows, fingers, and ankles occurred. Arthralgias worsened, morning stiffness was present, and her weight decreased from 59 to 41 kg. Painful buccal and palate ulcers developed simultaneously with a purpuric rash on the legs. She presented when she developed hoarseness and stridor.

Physical Examination: Temperature 98.6°; respirations 16; heart rate 80, regular; blood pressure 140/90. General: asthenic and hoarse. Skin: palpable purpuric skin lesions measuring 3–4 mm over the legs. HEENT: shallow erosions of the hard and soft palate. Neck: mild anterior tenderness without goiter or mass. Lungs: clear. Cardiac: normal. Abdomen: normal. Neurologic: normal. Musculoskeletal: no synovitis.

Laboratory Findings: Hct 34%; WBC 9,400/μL with normal differential; platelet count 495,000/μL. Chemistries: normal. ANA 1:640 with homogeneous pattern. Anti-DNA antibody: negative. C3 and C4: normal. Chest radiograph: normal. Skin biopsy: leukocytoclastic vasculitis. Direct laryngoscopy: thickened vocal cords fixed in midposition. Laryngeal tomograms: see Figure. Drug acetylator phenotype: slow.

Question: What is the diagnosis and the cause of the patient's hoarseness?

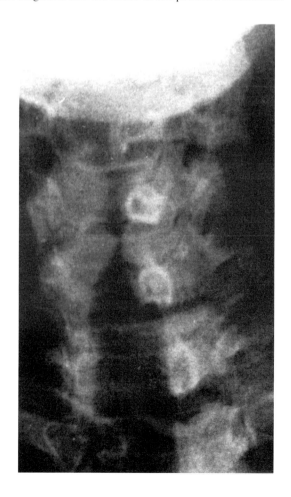

Diagnosis: Drug-induced lupus with laryngeal involvement (hydralazine hoarseness).

Discussion: A diagnosis of drug-induced lupus was made on the basis of arthralgias, oral ulcers, leukocytoclastic vasculitis, and high-titer ANA with homogeneous pattern in this elderly woman with a slow drug acetylator phenotype treated with increasing doses of hydralazine. Among the drugs that have definitely been associated with lupus are hydralazine, procainamide, chlorpromazine, methyldopa, and isoniazid. Other drugs possibly capable of inducing lupus include phenytoin, quinidine, and penicillamine. In many cases, the risk of developing drug-induced lupus appears to be related to drug acetylator phenotype. Patients who are slow acetylators develop ANAs sooner and clinical features consistent with lupus more rapidly than do patients who are fast acetylators. Nearly all patients with hydralazine-induced lupus are slow acetylators. Idiopathic SLE does not appear to be related to acetylator phenotype.

Clinical features of drug-induced lupus are generally less severe than those of SLE. The most commonly reported symptoms associated with drug-induced lupus are fever, weight loss, arthritis, and serositis. CNS and renal involvement are seen less commonly in drug-induced lupus than in idiopathic SLE, as are antibodies to DNA and hypocomplementemia. On the other hand, anti-histone antibodies are detected more commonly in drug-induced lupus than in idiopathic SLE. Various anti-histone profiles have been associated with different drugs.

An unusual feature in the present case was hoarseness and stridor with thickened vocal cords. Laryngeal involvement has rarely been described in drug-induced lupus and is often overlooked in idiopathic SLE. Common symptoms are hoarseness, dyspnea, and dysphagia. Involvement ranges from mild ulcerations, vocal cord paralysis, and edema to necrotizing vasculitis with airway obstruction. In the majority of cases, symptoms resolve with corticosteroid therapy. Life-threatening upper airway compromise may require urgent endotracheal intubation or tracheotomy. Other less common causes of laryngeal symptoms in lupus patients include subglottic stenosis, nodules, inflammatory mass lesions, necrotizing vasculitis, and epiglottitis.

In the present case hoarseness, constitutional symptoms, rash, and arthralgias resolved with prednisone, 60 mg daily, and discontinuation of hydralazine. Steroids were discontinued after 2 months and laryngoscopy was normal after 3 months. At 7 months, the ANA remained positive at a titer of 1:160.

Clinical Pearls

1. Drugs that are definitely associated with lupus include hydralazine, procainamide, chlorpromazine, and isoniazid.

2. Hydralazine-induced lupus is nearly always associated with a slow drug acetylator phenotype; idiopathic SLE does not appear to be related to drug acetylator phenotype.

3. Laryngeal involvement should be considered in the patient with idiopathic or with drug-induced lupus who complains of hoarseness, dysphagia, odynophagia, dyspnea, or stridor.

4. Most patients with drug-induced lupus improve within days or weeks after the offending drug is discontinued; a short course of corticosteroids may hasten improvement.

REFERENCES

1. Weiser GA, Forouhar FA, White WB. Hydralazine hoarseness. A new appearance of drug-induced systemic lupus erythematosus. Arch Intern Med 1984; 144:2271–2272.
2. Maxwell D, Silver R. Laryngeal manifestations of drug induced lupus. J Rheumatol 1987; 14:375–377.
3. Russell GI, Bing RF, Jones JA, Thurston H, Swales JD. Hydralazine sensitivity: clinical features, autoantibody changes and HLA-DR phenotype. Q J Med 1987; 65:845–852.
4. Teitel AD, Mackenzie CR, Stern R, Paget SA. Laryngeal involvement in systemic lupus erythematosus. Semin Arthritis Rheum 1992; 22:203–214.
5. Hess EV, Farhey Y. Epidemiology, genetics, etiology, and environment relationships of systemic lupus erythematosus. Curr Opin Rheumatol 1994; 6:474–480.

PATIENT 38

A 33-year-old woman with heel pain

A 33-year-old woman with a 1-year history of right heel pain was seen. She denied traumatic injury, but stated she worked in a textile mill on her feet for up to 14 hours daily. She had no other musculoskeletal complaints. She denied having a rash, eye inflammation, or dysuria. The patient remembered having a 3-week diarrheal illness before onset of the heel pain and still notes loose stools twice weekly. Her father had an inflammatory arthritis of the right elbow.

Physical Examination: Vital signs: normal. Skin: normal. HEENT: normal. Cardiopulmonary: normal. Abdomen: normal. Neurologic: normal. Musculoskeletal: thickened, tender right Achilles tendon with atrophy of the calf, pain on dorsiflexion and inversion of the right foot, and painful plantar fascia. Schöber index: normal.

Laboratory Findings: CBC: normal. Uric acid: normal. RF: negative. ANA: negative. Westergren ESR: 6 mm/hr. HLA B-27: positive. HIV: negative. Sacroiliac radiographs: normal. Ankle radiographs: small plantar spur and slight opacification of the pre-Achilles fat triangle suggestive of inflammation. MRI (shown below): increased signal intensity within the distal right Achilles tendon measuring 1.3 cm in transverse diameter.

Question: What is the cause and treatment of this patient's heel pain?

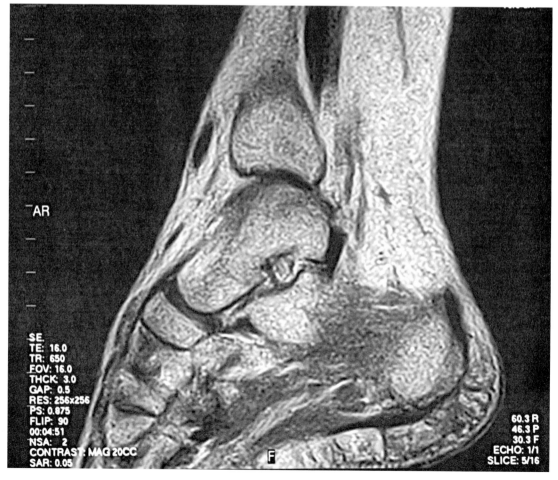

Diagnosis: Incomplete Reiter's syndrome.

Discussion: Reiter's syndrome classically refers to peripheral arthritis, nonspecific urethritis and conjunctivitis following a dysenteric illness or venereal disease. Reiter's syndrome is a reactive arthritis that occurs in a genetically susceptible host (HLA-B27 positive) following infection of the gut by Salmonella, Shigella, Yersinia, or Campylobacter, or of the genitourinary tract by Chlamydia. An incomplete form of Reiter's syndrome occurs as an asymmetric oligoarthritis of the lower extremities without urethritis or conjunctivitis.

One should consider the diagnosis of Reiter's syndrome in any patient with an asymmetric oligoarthritis involving lower extremity joints, especially if there is heel pain. Unlike rheumatoid arthritis, Reiter's syndrome is asymmetric and has a predilection for lower extremity joints. Patients with Reiter's syndrome are RF negative, and the ESR is often normal.

Occasional patients with long-standing Reiter's syndrome develop axial disease and, like patients with ankylosing spondylitis, have limited lumbar flexion and abnormal Schöber test. The Schöber test entails a measurement of 10 cm over the lumbar area with the patient erect. An increase of less than 5 cm when the patient is asked to touch the floor implies inability to reverse the lumbar lordosis and is often seen in patients with seronegative spondyloarthropathy.

Another feature of seronegative spondyloarthropathy, including Reiter's syndrome, is its tendency to cause inflammation at tendinous insertions into bone, *enthesopathy.* This gives rise to the "sausage digit" in the hands or feet, as well as to Achilles tendinitis and plantar fasciitis in the foot. Similar findings may be seen in the other HLA-B27 related conditions: ankylosing spondylitis, psoriatic arthritis, and inflammatory bowel disease.

Achilles tendinitis due to Reiter's syndrome gives rise to chronic hind foot swelling and pain (talalgia). Other causes of acute or chronic Achilles tendinitis include trauma, athletic overuse, RA, gout, pseudogout, xanthomas in hyperlipoproteinemias, and the other HLA-B27 associated conditions. The presence of heel pain often correlates with a poor prognosis and may lead to work disability.

Plain radiographs, ultrasound, and MRI may be useful to demonstrate Achilles tendinitis. In normal individuals the thickness of the Achilles tendon is between 4 and 8 mm at the level of the calcaneus. With inflammation, the tendon is thickened. An associated retrocalcaneal bursitis may obliterate the normal radiolucency that extends at least 2 mm below the posterosuperior surface of the calcaneus.

Treatment of Achilles tendinitis includes NSAIDs, heel support, splinting (ankle-foot orthosis), and gentle stretching. The Achilles tendon is vulnerable to rupture and must not be injected with corticosteroid, but retrocalcaneal bursitis and plantar fasciitis may respond to injected corticosteroid. Resistant cases may improve with sulfasalazine, methotrexate, or azathioprine. Reiter's disease may be the presenting manifestation of human immunodeficiency virus (HIV) infection. In such cases, it is usually incomplete with enthesopathy and fasciitis of the feet being dominant features. Immunosuppressive therapy is contraindicated in HIV-positive patients. Local radiotherapy to the heel may yield prompt and persistent improvement in cases refractory to conservative treatment.

In the present case, a diagnosis of incomplete Reiter's syndrome was made in this young woman who was HLA-B27 positive with Achilles tendinitis following a diarrheal illness. Ileocolonoscopy was negative for inflammatory bowel disease. Achilles tendinitis failed to respond to NSAIDs, orthotics, sulfasalazine, and methotrexate. Soft tissue swelling resolved with local radiotherapy, but pain and disability persisted.

Clinical Pearls

1. Talalgia, or heel pain, may be the first symptom of seronegative spondyloarthropathy: Reiter's syndrome, ankylosing spondylitis, psoriatic arthritis, inflammatory bowel disease.

2. Reiter's syndrome (arthritis, nonspecific urethritis, and conjunctivitis) may present with arthritis alone (incomplete Reiter's syndrome), in which case heel pain is usually a prominent feature.

3. Incomplete Reiter's syndrome, especially enthesopathy and fasciitis of the feet, may be a manifestation of human immunodeficiency virus (HIV) infection.

4. Heel pain secondary to Reiter's syndrome is often chronic and may be disabling.

5. Radiographic features of Reiter's syndrome involving the heel include thickening of the Achilles tendon, obliteration of the retrocalcaneal recess, ill-defined spurs, and/or erosions of the plantar and posterior aspects of the calcaneus.

6. Refractory cases of Achilles tendinitis may respond to a course of local radiotherapy.

REFERENCES

1. Smith DL, Bennett RM, Regan MG. Reiter's disease in women. Arthritis Rheum 1980;23:335–340.
2. Gerster JC, Sandan Y, Fallet GH. Talalgia. A review of 30 severe cases. J Rheumatol 1978;5:210–216.
3. Resnick D, Feingold ML, Curd J, Ninayama G, Goergen TG. Calcaneal abnormalities in articular disorders. Radiology 1977;125:355–366.
4. Fox R, Calin A, Gerber RC, Gibson D. The chronicity of symptoms and disability in Reiter's syndrome. An analysis of 131 consecutive patients. Ann Intern Med 1979;91:190–193.
5. Winchester R. AIDS and the rheumatic diseases. Bull Rheum Dis 1990;39(5):1–10.
6. Grill V, Smith M, Ahern M, Littlejohn G. Local radiotherapy for pedal manifestations of HLA- B27-related arthropathy. Br J Rheumatol 1988;27:390–392.

PATIENT 39

A 41-year-old woman with taut skin and cirrhosis

A 41-year-old woman presented with a 12-year history of scleroderma beginning as a plaque of taut skin on the chest spreading to involve other areas of the trunk and neck. She denied skin changes on the face or extremities, and symptoms of Raynaud's phenomenon. Recently, she was found to have elevated liver function tests but denied jaundice, pruritus, hepatitis, blood transfusion, or intravenous drug use. There was no history of sicca symptoms, photosensitivity, dysphagia, or dyspnea. She worked as a dental assistant.

Physical Examination: Vital signs: normal. Skin: multiple sclerotic hyperpigmented plaques on the abdomen, chest, back, and neck with sparing of the face, arms, and legs. HEENT: normal. Chest: clear. Cardiovascular: normal. Abdomen: mild splenomegaly. Neurologic: normal. Musculoskeletal: normal. Extremities: no cyanosis or acrosclerosis.

Laboratory Findings: WBC 7100/μL; Hct 41%; platelets 343,000/μL; serum electrolytes normal; AST 121 IU/L; ALT 176 IU/L; alkaline phosphatase 278 IU/L; bilirubin 0.8 mg/dL; ANA and antimitochondrial antibody (AMA) negative; anti-smooth muscle antibody positive, 1:20; serum protein electrophoresis normal; hepatitis serology negative; nailfold capillary microscopy normal; skin biopsy showed effacement of the rete ridges with expansion of dermis by thick collagen bundles, superficial and deep mononuclear cell perivascular infiltrate. Liver biopsy: see Figure.

Question: What is the diagnosis?

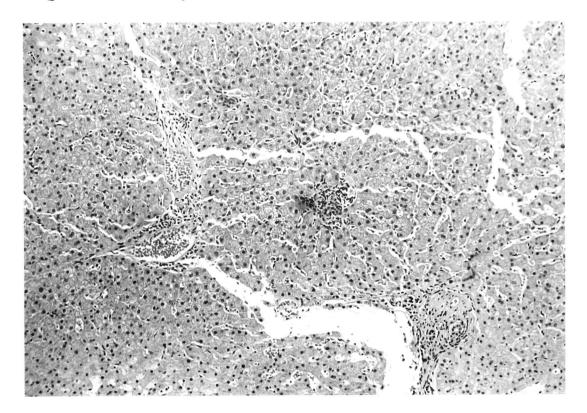

Diagnosis: Primary biliary cirrhosis with generalized morphea.

Discussion: Primary biliary cirrhosis (PBC) is an autoimmune disease characterized by lymphocytic infiltration and destruction of small bile ducts, often in association with antibodies and T cell clones with specificity for mitochondrial autoantigens. Extensive lymphocytic infiltration of the portal tracts may occur with varying degrees of bile duct damage, portal and bridging fibrosis, and in some cases cirrhosis (see Figure). A variety of autoimmune diseases have been associated with PBC, most frequently limited cutaneous systemic sclerosis (CREST syndrome) and Sjögren's syndrome, but also lupus, RA, and thyroiditis.

Up to 15% of patients with PBC have scleroderma, and most of these have the CREST variant with both antimitochondrial and anticentromere antibodies. Rarely, cases of localized scleroderma or generalized morphea, as in the present case, have been described. The histopathologic findings of mild epidermal atrophy with marked dermal thickening due to collagen accumulation and mononuclear cell infiltration is seen in both localized scleroderma (morphea) and systemic sclerosis, including the CREST syndrome. The absence of Raynaud's phenomena, acrosclerosis and esophageal dysmotility, plus the negative ANA and normal nailfold capillary morphology, established the diagnosis of morphea in the present patient with taut skin and characteristic dermatopathology. Other skin diseases occurring in association with PBC include lichen planus, pemphigoid, vitiligo, and lichen sclerosis et atrophicus.

At least three other women with indurated cutaneous plaques typical of morphea and histologic evidence of PBC have been reported. In one case the skin softened with oxypentifylline. Unlike the present patient, they were found to have antimitochondrial antibodies (AMA). Antimitochondrial antibodies of the M2 type are diagnostic of PBC and are mainly directed against an epitope of the pyruvate dehydrogenase complex. Since generalized morphea is one of the cutaneous manifestations of chronic graft-versus-host disease (GVHD), and PBC resembles the hepatic histology of chronic GVHD, the two conditions may have a common pathogenesis.

In the present case, the coexistence of PBC and generalized morphea was confirmed by liver and skin biopsy, respectively. PBC was treated with ursodeoxycholic acid and morphea was treated with hydroxychloroquine.

Clinical Pearls

1. Primary biliary cirrhosis (PBC) is an autoimmune liver disease characterized by lymphocytic destruction of small bile ducts, often with antibodies directed against mitochondrial antigens.

2. PBC may occur in association with other autoimmune conditions including scleroderma, Sjögren's syndrome, lupus, rheumatoid arthritis, and thyroiditis.

3. Approximately 15% of PBC patients have scleroderma, usually limited cutaneous systemic sclerosis (CREST syndrome), often with antimitochondrial (AMA) and anticentromere antibodies (ACA).

4. PBC may occur in association with localized scleroderma (generalized morphea).

5. Generalized morphea is identical histologically to systemic scleroderna, but is distinguished by the absence of acrosclerosis, Raynaud's phenomena or internal organ involvement, as well as the presence of normal nailfold capillary morphology.

REFERENCES

1. Natarajan S, Green ST. Generalized morphea, lichen sclerosus et atrophicus and primary biliary cirrhosis. Clin Exp Dermatol 1986;11:304–308.
2. Suyama Y, Murawaki Y, Horie Y, et al. A case of primary biliary cirrhosis associated with generalized morphea. Hepatogastroenterology 1986; 33:199–200.
3. Hirakata M, Akizuki M, Miyachi K, Matsushima H, Okano T, Homma M. Coexistence of CREST syndrome and primary biliary cirrhosis. Serological studies of two cases. J Rheumatol 1988; 15:1166–1170.
4. McMahon RFT, Babbs C, Warnes TW. Nodular regenerative hyperplasia of the liver, CREST syndrome and primary biliary cirrhosis: an overlap syndrome? Gut 1989; 30:1430–1433.
5. McHugh NJ, James IE, Fairburn K, Maddison PJ. Autoantibodies to mitochondrial and centromere antigens in primary biliary cirrhosis and systemic sclerosis. Clin Exp Immunol 1990; 81:244–249.
6. Wong SS, Holt PJA. Generalized morphoea and primary biliary cirrhosis: a rare association and improvement with oxypentifylline. Clin Exp Dermatol 1992; 17:371–373.
7. Whyte J, Hough D, Maddison PJ, McHugh NJ. The association of primary biliary cirrhosis and systemic sclerosis is not accounted for by cross reactivity between mitochondrial and centromere antigens. J Autoimmun 1994; 7:413–424.

PATIENT 40

A 47-year-old woman with hepatitis and rash

A 47-year-old woman had a 7-year history of an erythematous lower extremity skin rash. The skin lesions were chronic and intermittent, recurring every 2 to 3 weeks, and were exacerbated by dependency. She also reported leg edema, arthralgia, paresthesias, and weakness. She had a history of von Willebrand's disease complicated by postpartum hemorrhage 25 years earlier that required blood and cryoprecipitate transfusions. Six weeks later, she became jaundiced. The jaundice resolved, but liver tests remained abnormal.

Physical Examination: Vital signs: normal. Skin: palpable purpuric lesions over the legs and feet. HEENT: normal. Chest: clear. Cardiovascular: normal. Abdomen: no ascites or hepatosplenomegaly. Neurologic: decreased sensation in lower extremities. Musculoskeletal: normal.

Laboratory Findings: WBC 3700 cells/μL; Hct 37.1%; platelets 172,000/μL; electrolytes normal; LDH 127 IU/L; AST 24 IU/L; ALT 14 IU/L; alkaline phosphatase 70 IU/L; total bilirubin 1.6 mg/dL; GGT 19 U/L; hepatitis B surface antigen and antibody negative; hepatitis C RIBA positive; hepatitis C quantitative viral RNA 14.3×10^5 eq/mL (limit of detection: 3.5×10^5 eq/mL); ESR 21 mm/hr; ANA negative; RF positive, 170 IU/mL; C3 76.6 mg/dL; C4 12.9 mg/dL; cryoglobulin 63 mg/dL, containing IgG, IgA, IgM and C1q; urinalysis normal. Nerve conduction velocity: severe peripheral neuropathy. Liver biopsy: see Figure.

Question: What is the diagnosis and treatment?

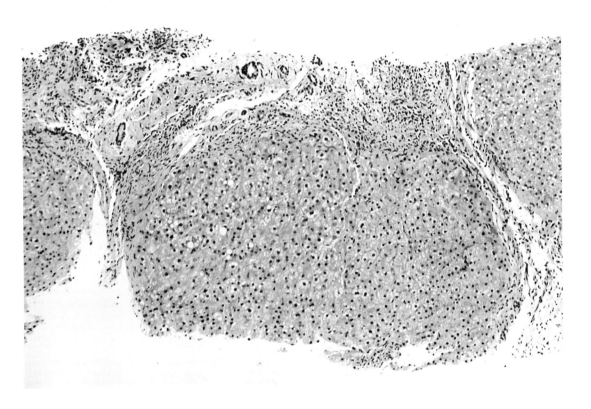

Diagnosis: Mixed cryoglobulinemia with hepatitis C virus infection.

Discussion: Cryoglobulins are cold-precipitable immunoproteins present in the serum of patients with a variety of diseases. Cryoglobulins may consist of a single monoclonal immunoglobulin (type I), as in Waldenström's macroglobulinemia and multiple myeloma, or as polyclonal (mixed) immunoglobulins in infections, autoimmune diseases, lymphoproliferative disorders, or in "essential mixed cryoglobulinemia" (when no underlying disease is found). Mixed cryoglobulins contain either monoclonal IgM RF (type II) or polyclonal IgM (type III).

Essential mixed cryoglobulinemia is seen most commonly in middle-aged women. The classic symptoms are purpura, arthralgia, and weakness. Palpable purpura occurs most commonly on the lower extremities. Biopsy reveals a leukocytoclastic vasculitis of the dermal vessels. Polyarthralgia is symmetric and not associated with erosive arthritis. Weakness may be profound. Peripheral neuropathy leads to lower extremity paresthesias and numbness and may be the presenting symptom. Other, less common, clinical manifestations include renal disease, Sjögren's syndrome, Raynaud's phenomenon, and skin ulcers.

Hepatitis is now recognized as a frequent and perhaps primary aspect of mixed cryoglobulinemia. Initial studies found a variable association between hepatitis B virus infection and essential mixed cryoglobulinemia. Recent studies using sensitive and specific markers of hepatitis C virus (HCV) infection, e.g., PCR, have established a clear association of HCV with mixed cryoglobulinemia. The prevalence of HCV antibody in serum for patients with mixed cryoglobulinema ranges from 30% to 98%, depending in part on the sensitivity of the method of detection. HCV RNA is detectable in serum of many patients. HCV antibody is concentrated in some cryoprecipitates. Other rheumatic manifestations of viral hepatitis include an acute, self-limited polyarthritis and polyarteritis nodosa.

The presence of HCV RNA in sera and cryoprecipitates supports the use of interferon alfa and other antiviral drugs in the treatment of HCV-associated mixed cryoglobulinemia. Treatment may reduce the level of circulating HCV RNA below the level of detection, with concomitant improvement in clinical and laboratory parameters. Viremia and cryoglobulinemia may recur where interferon-alfa is discontinued. Patients must be monitored for leukopenia and thrombocytopenia while receiving interferon-alfa therapy.

In the present patient with palpable purpura, weakness, polyarthralgia, and peripheral neuropathy, a diagnosis of mixed cryoglobulinemia with chronic hepatitis C infection was made. Liver biopsy confirmed the presence of chronic hepatitis and cirrhosis (see Figure), despite normal serum transaminase levels. Treatment with interferon-alfa was accompanied by improvement in nerve conduction velocity, rash, and weakness, with a fall in cryoglobulinemia. Mild leukopenia and thrombocytopenia necessitated reduction in interferon-alfa.

Clinical Pearls

1. Cryoglobulins of the mixed type occur in various infections, autoimmune diseases and lymphoproliferative disorders or without an underlying disease (essential mixed cryoglobulinemia).

2. Consider the diagnosis of cryoglobulinema in the patient with palpable purpura, weakness, and arthralgia.

3. Small-vessel vasculitis secondary to cryoglobulinema may produce peripheral neuropathy, which may be the presenting manifestation.

4. A high proportion of patients with so-called essential mixed cryoglobulinema have evidence of chronic hepatitis C virus infection.

5. Significant improvement in symptoms and a decrease in cryoglobulinema may occur with interferon-alfa therapy.

REFERENCES

1. Levo Y, Gorevic PD, Kassub HJ, et al. Association between hepatitis B virus and essential mixed cryoglobulinema. N Engl J Med 1977; 296:1501–1504.
2. Abel G, Zhang QX, Agnello V. Hepatitis C infection in type II mixed cryoglobulins. Arthritis Rheum 1993;98:1341–1349.
3. Levey JM, Bjornsson B, Banner B, et al. Mixed cryoglobulinemia in chronic hepatitis C infection. A clinicopathologic analysis of 10 cases and review of the literature. Medicine (Baltimore) 1994; 73:53–67.
4. Misiani R, Bellavita P, Fevili D, et al. Interferon alfa-2a therapy in cryoglobulinema associated with hepatitis C virus. N Engl J Med 1994; 330:751–756.

PATIENT 41

A 60-year-old man with arthritis, hypertension, and anemia

A 60-year-old man presented with acute swelling, warmth, and pain involving the right ankle and knee. He reported similar self-limited, monoarticular attacks over the past 5 years, usually involving the great toe or instep. Past medical history was remarkable for alcohol abuse, including moonshine.

Physical Examination: Vital signs: temperature 99.6°, pulse 80, respirations 16, blood pressure 160/110. Skin: nontender, subcutaneous olecranon bursal nodules and chalky deposits in helix of ears. HEENT: arteriolar narrowing. Chest: clear. Cardiac: S4 gallop. Abdomen: normal. Neurologic: normal. Musculoskeletal: effusions of right knee and ankle with decreased flexion and surrounding warmth and erythema.

Laboratory Findings: WBC 10,500/μL; Hct 32%; platelets 160,000/μL; serum potassium: 5 mmol/L; serum creatinine 1.9 mg/dL; serum uric acid 10.9 mg/dL; urinalysis: 2+proteinuria, 10–20 leukocytes/hpf, 5–10 RBC/hpf; urine culture: negative; foot radiographs: soft tissue swelling with erosions at the first MTP joints and overhanging rim of sclerotic bone; synovial fluid analysis: WBC 55,000/μL with 85% neutrophils, 15% monocytes, glucose 60 mg/dL, negatively birefringent, needle-shaped, intracellular crystals on polarizing microscopy (see Figure).

Question: What test confirms the etiology of this patient's tophaceous gout?

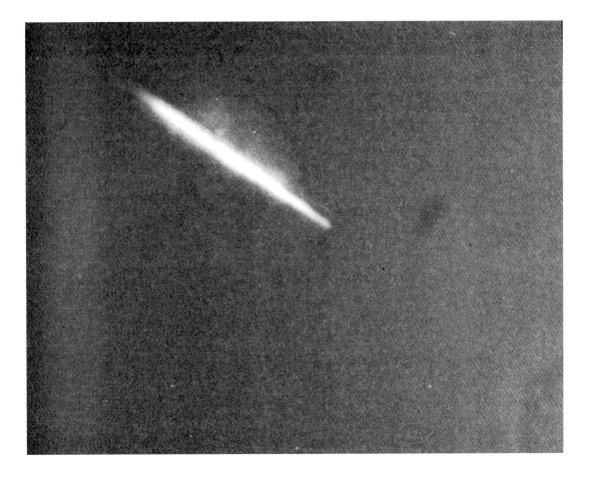

Diagnosis: Saturnine gout confirmed by EDTA lead mobilization test.

Discussion: The deposition of monosodium urate crystals from supersaturated extracellular fluids results in a number of clinical manifestations, including acute or chronic arthritis; tophi; nephrolithiasis. All stem from hyperuricemia (> 7.0 mg/dL), which is the result of uric acid overproduction or uric acid underexcretion. The majority of patients with primary hyperuricemia and gout have a relative impairment in renal excretion of uric acid.

Chronic lead nephropathy often leads to hyperuricemia and gout due to slowly progressive renal failure with tubulointerstitial disease and nephrosclerosis. Associated complications include hypertension, anemia, and hyperkalemia (type IV RTA). Sources of chronic lead poisoning include occupational lead exposure (e.g., smelting, solder manufacturing, painting) and ingestion of illicit alcohol (moonshine). Moonshine is often contaminated with lead if radiators containing lead-soldered connections are used as condensers, or if lead plates are added by the distiller to "improve" the taste of the liquor.

There is a long history of lead-induced or "saturnine" gout resulting from drinking lead-contaminated alcohol. In the eighteenth and nineteenth centuries, lead-contaminated wines were associated with an "epidemic" of gout in England. Saturnine gout is now recognized as a complication of chronic moonshine indulgence, particularly among black males in the southeastern United States.

Unlike acute lead poisoning, routine blood and urine samples do not reflect chronic lead poisoning. Lead is stored in bone, and the diagnostic test for chronic lead poisoning is measurement of urinary lead excretion following chelation with edentate calcium disodium (calcium EDTA). EDTA is given IM or IV at a dose of 25 mg/kg not to exceed 1.0 gm. Urine is collected for 24 hours if renal function is normal, or for 72 hours if renal function is impaired since renal insufficiency delays excretion of lead chelate during the EDTA test. A finding of 600 μg or more of lead during the collection period is diagnostic of lead poisoning (plumbism).

Therapy of saturnine gout does not differ from other forms of chronic tophaceous gout. Acute gouty attacks are treated with colchicine, NSAIDs and/or intra-articular corticosteroid. Allopurinol may be added later to colchicine, titrating the dose to lower the serum uric acid to 7 mg/dL or less. If renal insufficiency is present, daily doses of allopurinol less than 300 mg may be sufficient. Chelation therapy, while beneficial in acute lead poisoning, may not be as effective in the chronic condition, and can cause side-effects, e.g., hypotension, hypocalcemia, thrombophlebitis, and acute renal failure.

In the present case, gout was diagnosed by the presence of monosodium urate crystals in synovial fluid, together with tophi, hyperuricemia, and classic radiographic erosions. With the history of moonshine ingestion, saturnine gout was suspected. Saturnine gout was confirmed by an EDTA lead mobilization test showing 850 μg lead/72-hour urine collection. Acute gout responded to intra-articular corticosteroid, and chronic hyperuricemia resolved with allopurinol; hypertension, anemia, and azotemia persisted.

Clinical Pearls

1. The majority of patients with primary hyperuricemia and gout have a relative impairment in renal excretion of uric acid.

2. Chronic lead poisoning leads to progressive renal failure with tubulointerstitial disease and nephrosclerosis and may present as gouty arthritis.

3. Consider the diagnosis of "saturnine gout" in the gouty patient with renal insufficiency, hypertension, and anemia, plus a history of moonshine ingestion or occupational lead exposure.

4. Lead is stored in bone and, unlike acute poisoning, blood lead levels may not reflect chronic intoxication.

5. Confirm the diagnosis of chronic lead poisoning with the EDTA lead mobilization test (> 600 μg lead/72 hours).

REFERENCES

1. Emmerson BT. Chronic lead nephropathy: The diagnostic use of calcium EDTA and the association with gout. Aust Ann Med 1963; 12:310–323.
2. Halla JT and Ball GV. Saturnine gout: A review of 42 cases. Semin Arthritis Rheum 1982; 11:307–314.
3. Batuman V. Lead nephropathy, gout and hypertension. Am J Med Sci 1993; 305:241–247.

PATIENT 42

An 81-year-old woman with dysphagia and malnutrition

An 81-year-old woman was admitted to the hospital for evaluation of dysphagia accompanied by a 20-pound weight loss. Symptoms began a year earlier with a sore throat that resolved but was followed by dysphagia for solid foods. Past history was remarkable for carcinoma of the colon, hypertension, congestive heart failure, osteoarthritis, and osteoporosis. The latter was complicated by compression fracture of the T8 vertebral body with secondary kyphosis and scoliosis.

Physical examination: Temperature 98.2°; pulse 96, respirations 24, blood pressure 180/120. Weight 94 lbs; height 61.5 inches. General appearance: cachectic woman in no acute distress. Skin: normal. Lymph nodes: normal. HEENT: atrophic glossitis. Neck: no goiter; reversal of cervical curve. Back: kyphoscoliosis. Chest: moist crackles. Cardiovascular: cardiomegaly with grade III/VI holosystolic murmur. Abdomen: normal. Neurologic: normal. Musculoskeletal: no peripheral joint deformities.

Laboratory findings: WBC 10,700/μL; Hct 43.9%; platelets 280,000/μL. Electrolytes: normal. Liver function tests: normal. Urinalysis: normal. ESR 6 mm/hr; RF negative; thyroid panel normal. Chest radiograph: cardiomegaly, calcified unfolded aorta and interstitial pulmonary edema. Esophagram: tertiary esophageal contractions. EGD: normal. Echocardiogram: concentric left ventricular hypertrophy, dilated left atrium, and sclerotic aortic valve. Cervical spine: see Figure.

Question: What is the cause of this patient's dysphagia?

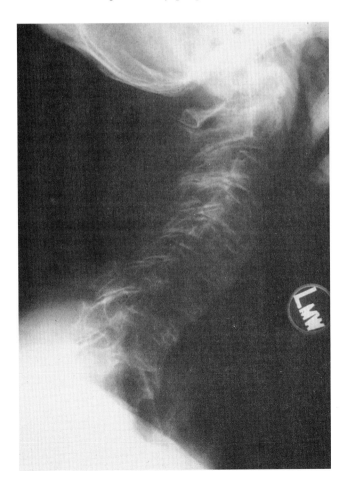

Diagnosis: Cervical spondylitic dysphagia.

Discussion: Impingement of the esophagus by cervical osteophytes may lead to dysphagia. Mechanical compression with or without inflammation of the adjacent soft tissue may produce symptoms of dysphagia, sometimes of sudden onset. If laryngotracheal compression accompanies esophageal involvement, it may lead to dyspnea, dysphonia, obstructive sleep apnea or cough, as well as dysphagia.

Hypertrophic changes of the cervical vertebrae occur commonly in cervical spondylosis, as in the present case, or in ankylosing hyperostosis. The latter, also known as diffuse idiopathic skeletal hyperostosis (DISH) or "Forestier disease" is a noninflammatory disease characterized by extensive bone formation and bridging vertebral osteophytes. Dysphagia occurs in 17% of patients with DISH, due to impingement of the esophagus by cervical osteophytes. Dysphagia may rarely occur due to exostosis arising from a cervical vertebra.

The absence of dysphagia in some patients with cervical osteophytes may be explained by the mobility of the esophagus. The esophagus is fixed at only two points: at the level of the cricoid cartilage and at the diaphragm. A large anterior osteophyte at either of these two relatively immobile points might result in dysphagia.

Barium swallow examination, indirect laryngoscopy, neurologic investigation, and EGD may all be normal but should be performed to exclude other causes of dysphagia. Cine-esophagram may show a partial hold-up of contrast in the midcervical region. Lateral cervical spine radiographs may show anterior osteophytes with disc space narrowing and apophyseal joint disease in patients with cervical spondylosis, or bridging osteophytes with normal disc height and apophyseal joints in patients with DISH. Radiographs of patients with DISH may also demonstrate ossification of the anterior and/or posterior longitudinal ligament.

Treatment by surgical excision of the osteophytic bone may completely eliminate symptoms of dysphagia or obstructive sleep apnea. In the present case, complicating medical illness precluded surgical excision of the osteophyte. A percutaneous endoscopic gastrostomy tube was placed to allow adequate nutritional intake.

Clinical Pearls

1. Neurologic, neoplastic, or extrinsic conditions affecting the esophagus may produce dysphagia.

2. Consider cervical spondylitic dysphagia in patients with normal neurologic examinations and negative endoscopic studies who present with acute or chronic dysphagia.

3. Large anterior cervical osteophytes in patients with cervical spondylosis or in patients with diffuse idiopathic skeletal hyperostosis (DISH) may compress the esophagus, producing dysphagia, dysphonia, or obstructive sleep apnea.

4. Severe cases may be cured by surgical resection of the osteophyte.

REFERENCES

1. Oga M, Mashima T, Iwakuma T, Sugioka Y. Dysphagia complications in ankylosing spinal hyperostosis and ossification of the posterior longitudinal ligament. Roentgenographic findings of the developmental process of cervical osteophytes causing dysphagia. Spine 1993; 18:391–394.
2. Barros TE, Oliveira RP, Taricco MA, Gonzalez CH. Heriditary multiple exostoses and cervical ventral protuberance causing dysphagia. Spine 1995; 20:1640–1642.
3. Kodama M, Sawada H, Udaka F, Kameyama M, Koyama T. Dysphagia caused by an anterior cervical osteophyte: case report. Neuroradiology 1995; 37:58–59.
4. Hughes TA, Wiles CM, Lawrie BW, Smith AP. Case report: dysphagia and sleep apnoea associated with cervical osteophytes due to diffuse idiopathic skeletal hyperostosis (DISH). J Neurol Neurosurg Psychiatry 1994; 57:384.
5. Krause P, Castro WH. Cervical hyperostosis: a rare cause of dysphagia. Case description and bibliographical survey. Eur Spine J 1994; 3:56–58.
6. Kodama M, Sawada H, Udaka F, Kameyama M, Koyama T. Dysphagia caused by an anterior cervical osteophyte: case report. Neuroradiology 1995; 37:58–59.

PATIENT 43

An 86-year-old man with chronic foot pain

An 86-year-old man presented with a 6-month history of right foot pain. Pain was present only with weight bearing, causing him to discontinue walking. Previously he had walked 2.5 miles daily. His past history was remarkable only for hypertension treated with a diuretic. He had undergone bunionectomy of the left foot but denied trauma to the right foot.

Physical examination: Temperature 97.8°, pulse 80, respirations 18, blood pressure 160/90. Skin: normal. Lymph nodes: normal. HEENT: atherosclerotic retinal vasculature. Neck: no bruit. Chest: clear. Heart: normal. Abdomen: normal. Neurologic: decreased sensation to light touch, pinprick and thermal sensation below the knees, markedly decreased joint position sense in the toes, normal in the fingers, absent ankle jerks. Musculoskeletal: warmth and swelling over dorsum of right midfoot with collapsed plantar arch and normal ankle motion.

Laboratory findings: WBC 8,000/µL; Hct 41.5%; platelets 249,000/µL; Na$^+$ 140 mmol/L; K$^+$ 3.5 mmol/L; Cl$^-$ 98 mmol/L; CO$_2$ 32 mmol/L; BUN 28 mg/dL; glucose 139 mg/dL; creatinine 1.3 mg/dL; calcium 9.6 mg/dL. Synovial fluid analysis: yellow, cloudy; WBC 11 cells/µL with 33% neutrophils, 7% lymphocytes, 60% macrophages; glucose 90 mg/dL; urate and CPPD crystals absent. STS: negative. Foot radiograph: healed fractures at midshaft of 2nd and 3rd metatarsals with evidence of old Lisfranc's fracture and osteoarthritic changes involving the tarsal bones. Technetium-MDP bone scan (shown below): increased activity on flow, immediate and delayed images of right foot.

Question: What is the diagnosis?

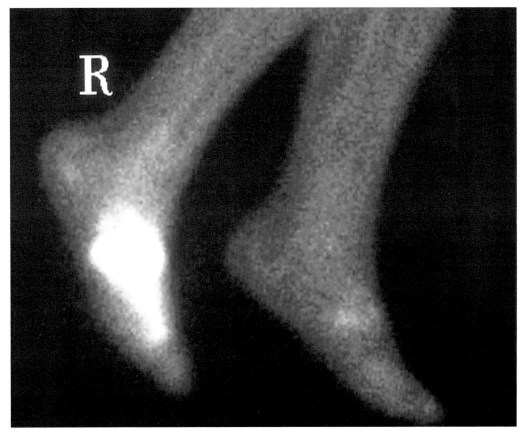

Diagnosis: Diabetic neuroarthropathy (Charcot joint).

Discussion: Charcot described the association of certain arthropathies with neurologic diseases—primarily tabes dorsalis—and the term "Charcot joint" is now applied to most articular abnormalities related to neurologic deficits. The terms neuroarthropathy and neutrophic and neuropathic joint disease are synonymous with Charcot joint. Neuropathy leads to loss of protective sensations of pain and proprioception which, in turn, lead to recurrent joint injury, malalignment, and progressive degeneration of the articulation.

Lesions of the central or peripheral nervous systems can lead to neuroarthropathy. Examples include syphilis (tabes dorsalis), syringomyelia, meningomyelocele, traumatic spine lesions, Charcot-Marie-Tooth disease, diabetes mellitus, alcoholism, pernicious anemia, and intra-articular administration of steroids. The distribution of the articular involvement varies among the neurologic disorders and may be a clue to diagnosis. Tabes dorsalis, complicated by neuroarthropathy in 5 to 10% cases, most commonly involves the knee, hip, ankle, or spine. Syringomyelia affects the shoulder, elbow, wrist, or spine. Alcoholism affects the foot and toes.

Diabetes mellitus is now a more frequent cause of neuroarthropathy than is syphilis. Neuroarthropathy has been noted in 0.15% of hospitalized diabetic patients, but the true incidence may be greater. Typically, diabetic neuroarthropathy occurs in the patient with long-standing diabetes mellitus. Occasionally, as in the present case, neuroarthropathy may be the initial clinical manifestation of diabetes mellitus. The joints in the forefoot and midfoot are most commonly affected, although the ankle, knee, spine, and joints of the upper extremities also can be affected.

Osseous fragmentation, sclerosis and subluxation or dislocation occur in the intertarsal or tarsometatarsal joints. The radiographic findings in the foot may resemble an acute Lisfranc's fracture-dislocation in which fracture at the base of the metatarsals (2nd–5th) and cuboid is associated with lateral dislocation of the 2nd through 5th metatarsal bones. Scintigraphy with bone-seeking radionuclides shows areas of increased accumulation of the radionuclide.

Bony eburnation, fracture, subluxation, and joint disorganization are more profound in neuroarthropathy than in any other arthropathy. Early cases may resemble osteoarthritis. Calcium pyrophosphate dihydrate crystal deposition (CPPD) disease can resemble neuroarthropathy, or may coexist with neuroarthropathy. Similar destructive changes may occur in the shoulder with calcium hydroxyapatite crystal deposition. Osteomyelitis, particularly in the diabetic foot, may mimic or be superimposed on a neuroarthropathy. An [111]indium-labeled white blood cell scan may help differentiate infected from noninfected rapidly progressive neuroarthropathy.

Treatment includes discerning the underlying cause of neuropathy. Diabetic neuroarthropathy of the foot may respond to a total-contact cast or brace. Some cases improve with arthrodesis; those that fail may require amputation.

In the present case, a diagnosis of diabetic foot neuroarthropathy was based on the presence of distal sensory neuropathy, hyperglycemia, and characteristic radiographic and scintigraphic changes. The patient had only a partial response to a molded orthotic insert and medical management of the diabetes mellitus.

Clinical Pearls

1. Neuroarthropathy, or Charcot joint, may occur in association with a variety of central or peripheral nervous system diseases.

2. Tabes dorsalis, once the most frequent cause of neuroarthropathy, generally affects the knee, hip, ankle or spine.

3. Diabetes mellitus is now the most frequent underlying cause of neuroarthropathy, usually affecting the joints of the forefoot and midfoot.

4. Neuroarthropathy is occasionally the initial clinical manifestation of diabetes mellitus.

5. Consider the diagnosis in the patient with sensory neuropathy and radiographs showing osseous fragmentation, sclerosis, subluxation, or dislocation with joint disorganization.

REFERENCES

1. Resnick D. Neuroarthropathy, In: Resnick D, Niwayama G (eds). Diagnosis of Bone and Joint Disorders. Philadelphia, WB Saunders 1988, pp 3154–3187.
2. Papa J, Myerson M, Girard P. Salvage, with arthrodesis, in intractable diabetic neuropathic arthropathy of the foot and ankle. J Bone Joint Surg (Am) 1993; 75:1056–1066.
3. Pedersen LM, Madsen OR, Bliddal H. Charcot arthropathy as an unusual initial manifestation of diabetes mellitus. Br J Rheumatol 1993; 32:854–855.
4. Myerson MS, Henderson MR, Saxby T, Short KW. Management of midfoot diabetic neuroarthropathy. Foot Ankle Int 1994; 15:233–241.
5. Sequeira W. The neuropathic joint. Clin Exp Rheumatol 1994; 12:325–337.
6. Schauweeker DS. Differentiation of infected from noninfected rapidly progressive neuropathic osteoarthropathy. J Nucl Med 1995; 36:1427–1428.

PATIENT 44

A 14-year-old girl with juvenile rheumatoid arthritis, painful wrists, and a weak thumb

A 14-year-old girl presented with chronic left wrist pain and acute thumb weakness. At age 11, she had an insidious onset of a symmetric polyarthritis involving small and large joints of the upper and lower extremities. A diagnosis of juvenile rheumatoid arthritis (JRA) was made. She was treated with NSAIDs, low-dose prednisone, hydroxychloroquine, and weekly low-dose oral methotrexate. She improved with treatment but continued to have bilateral wrist pain. She presented with a 1-day history of left thumb weakness.

Physical Examination: Temperature 98.9°, heart rate 90, respirations 18, blood pressure 90/60. Skin: no rash or subcutaneous nodules. Lymph nodes: normal. HEENT: normal. Neck: full ROM. Back: nontender. Chest: clear. Cardiac: normal. Abdomen: normal. Neurologic: normal. Musculoskeletal: fusiform swelling around the PIP joints of the fingers and IP joint of the thumbs; inability to extend the left thumb; mild synovitis on the dorsum of both wrists with full ROM; small, nontender effusion of left knee with full ROM.

Laboratory Findings: WBC 5,500/μL; Hct 35.8%; platelets 421,000/μL. ESR 65 mm/hr. RF: positive, 1:40 titer. ANA: positive, 1:160 titer, speckled. Anti-DNA antibody: negative. Serum chemistries: normal. Liver panel: normal. Left wrist radiograph (shown below): diffuse osteopenia, erosions of the capitate, collapse of the scaphoid and delayed development of the radial epiphysis.

Question: What is the cause of thumb weakness?

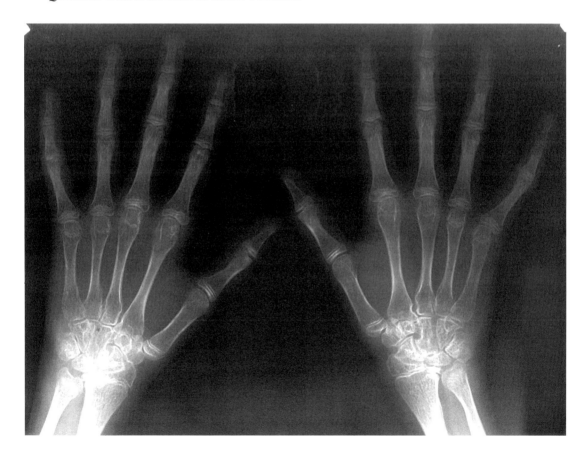

Diagnosis: JRA with rupture of the extensor pollicis longus tendon.

Discussion: An important subgroup of children with polyarticular JRA—accounting for approximately 5% all cases of JRA—includes girls who have onset of disease late in childhood or adolescence and are rheumatoid factor (RF)-positive. Children in other subtypes of JRA are nearly always RF-negative. Children in the seropositive (RF+) subset have a disease with clinical, radiographic, and immunogenetic features identical to adult-onset, RF-positive RA. These children are more prone to develop erosive synovitis, extra-articular manifestations, e.g., nodules, and a chronic course compared to children with other JRA subtypes.

Tenosynovitis occurs in up to 20% of children with JRA. The most common sites of tenosynovitis are the extensor tendon sheath over the dorsum of the hand, the flexor tendon sheath on the palmar aspect of the hand, the extensor sheath over the dorsum of the foot, and the posterior tibial, peroneus longus and brevis tendons around the ankle. A rare complication in children and adults with RA is stenosing tenosynovitis of the superior oblique tendon in the trochlea of the eye, presenting with diplopia upon upward gaze (Brown syndrome). Brown syndrome also occurs rarely in lupus and scleroderma.

Although dorsal (wrist) sheath swelling is not uncommon in children with JRA, extensor tendon rupture is rare. Only rarely has rupture of the extensor tendons to the fingers or the extensor pollicis longus been reported. Rupture occurs from attrition of the tendon by the proliferative synovitis, actual invasion of the tendon by pannus, and trauma to the tendon as it passes around Lister's tubercle on the distal radius.

Treatment of persistent tenosynovitis involves local corticosteroid injections. In resistant cases, or if rupture occurs, the patient should be referred immediately to a hand surgeon. Tenosynovectomy and, in the case of rupture, a tendon transfer may restore function of the tendon.

In the present case, an extensor tenosynovectomy was performed with a tendon transfer to restore function of the extensor pollicis longus. She recovered full range of motion and was able to resume playing the clarinet in her school band.

Clinical Pearls

1. The three major subtypes of JRA are defined by the type of disease in the first 6 months: (1) oligoarticular; (2) polyarticular; (3) systemic.

2. Only 5% of children with JRA are RF-positive, usually girls with onset of disease in late childhood or adolescence.

3. RF-positive JRA is similar to adult-onset RA in terms of clinical, radiographic, and immunogenetic features.

4. Tenosynovitis in JRA occurs most commonly in the extensor tendons on the dorsum of the hand, flexor tendons on the palmar aspect of the hand, extensor tendons on the dorsum of the foot and around the ankle.

5. Rupture of tendons due to JRA or RA requires immediate surgical consultation.

REFERENCES

1. Cassidy JT, Levinson JE, Bass JC, et al. A study of classification criteria for a diagnosis of juvenile rheumatoid arthritis. Arthritis Rheum 1986; 29:274–281.
2. Barnett AJ, Griffiths JC, West RH. Acquired Brown's syndrome. Ann Rheum Dis 1993; 52:835.
3. Juvenile rheumatoid arthritis. In: Cassidy JT and Petty RE (eds). Textbook of Pediatric Rheumatology. Philadelphia, WB Saunders, 1995, pp 133–223.
4. Williamson SC, Feldon P: Extensor tendon ruptures in rheumatoid arthritis. Hand Clin 1995; 11:449–459.

PATIENT 45

A 39-year-old man with vasculitis and neck pain

A 39-year-old man presented with fever, hypertension, arthralgia, and myalgia. Biopsy of a 4 cm ×
2 cm nodule in the right calf revealed necrotizing vasculitis involving medium-sized muscular arteries. A
diagnosis of polyarteritis nodosum (PAN) was established, and he was treated with cyclophosphamide, 2
mg/kg daily. His symptoms resolved, and cyclophosphamide was discontinued after 2 years. He presented
again 3 years later with a 2-week history of left-sided headache and neck pain made worse by changes in
head position, but not associated with vision changes, nausea, or vomiting.

Physical Examination: Temperature 98.6°; heart rate 80; respiratory rate 14; blood pressure 120/80
mmHg. Skin: no rash or nodules. Lymph nodes: negative. HEENT: normal. Neck: tender left carotid artery
underneath the mandible, no bruit. Back: normal. Chest: clear. Cardiac: normal. Abdomen: normal. Neurologic: normal. Musculoskeletal: normal. Extremities: normal.

Laboratory Findings: WBC 10,500/μL; Hct 37.5%; platelets 325,000/μL. ESR 72 mm/hr. Serum
chemistries: normal. Liver tests: normal. Urinalysis: normal. Chest radiograph: normal. ECG: normal.
Cerebrospinal fluid: normal. Carotid arteriogram (shown below).

Question: What is the cause of the neck pain?

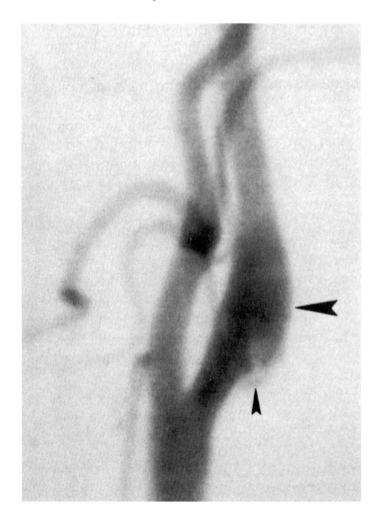

Answer: PAN with dissecting aneurysm of the left internal carotid artery.

Discussion: Polyarteritis nodosa (PAN) is a necrotizing vasculitis affecting small and medium-sized blood vessels. Patients often present with constitutional symptoms such as fever, night sweats, and weight loss. Hypertension is frequently present and associated with renal artery involvement. Mesenteric vasculitis, if present, causes postprandial abdominal pain (mesenteric angina) and may be complicated by mesenteric infarction or perforation. Other symptoms and signs occur depending on the extent and degree of vasculitis. A characteristic feature of PAN is aneurysmal dilatation of medium-sized arteries visible on angiography.

Large vessel involvement may also be present in patients with PAN. Aneurysmal dilatation with dissection of the internal carotid artery can occur, as in the present case, with unilateral headache and neck pain. Other causes of unilateral neck pain over the carotid artery—carotidynia—include migraine, pharyngitis or postinfection, giant cell arteritis, carotid artery aneurysm, dissection, or occlusion.

Most cases of internal carotid artery dissection occur spontaneously. Frequent presentations include headache, carotidynia, bruits, and oculosympathetic paresis. Complete Horner syndrome, tinnitus, dysgeusia, and involvement of cranial nerves V, VII, X, and XII, along with symptoms consistent with transient ischemic attacks and hemiplegia,

have been reported with internal carotid artery dissection. Diagnosis is confirmed by arteriography. Common arteriographic findings include irregular arterial narrowing (due to subintimal hemorrhage), which if severe and extensive results in the "string sign." Dissection usually begins distal to the origin of the internal carotid, where an intimal flap may be seen.

PAN may also lead to aortic dissection, in some cases due to necrotizing vasculitis of the vasa vasorum. More common causes of aortic dissection include atherosclerosis, cystic medial necrosis, hypertension, trauma, and syphilis. Giant cell arteritis—either temporal arteritis or Takayasu's arteritis—may also result in aortic dissection.

Neurologic sequelae of internal carotid artery dissections are due predominantly to thromboembolic events, rather than flow limitation alone. Patients should be anticoagulated to prevent cerebral embolization, and a search should be made for an underlying cause of the dissection.

The present patient was anticoagulated and treated with high-dose prednisone (20 mg tid) and daily oral cyclophosphamide (1.5 mg/kg). Within 1 week he was asymptomatic and the ESR was 17 mm/hr. Prednisone was tapered and discontinued, and oral anticoagulation was continued for 4 months. Cyclophosphamide was continued for 2 years.

Clinical Pearls

1. Polyarteritis nodosa (PAN) is a necrotizing vasculitis involving small and medium-sized muscular arteries.

2. A characteristic feature of PAN is aneurysmal dilatation of medium-sized arteries visible on angiography.

3. PAN may rarely involve large arteries, such as the internal carotid and the aorta.

4. Consider arteritis—either PAN or giant cell arteritis—in patients with carotidynia, internal carotid dissection, or aortic dissection.

5. Treatment of PAN consists of high-dose steroids and cyclophosphamide.

REFERENCES

1. Lomeo RM, Silver RM, Brothers M. Spontaneous dissection of the internal carotid artery in a patient with polyarteritis nodosa. Arthritis Rheum 1989; 32:1625–1626.
2. Iino T, Eguchi K, Sakai M, et al. Polyarteritis nodosa with aortic dissection: necrotizing vasculitis of the vasa vasorum. J Rheumatol 1992; 19:1632–1636.
3. Cannon CR. Carotidynia: An unusual pain in the neck. Otolaryngol Head Neck Surg 1994; 110:387–390.
4. Hill LM, Hastings G: Carotidynia: A pain syndrome. J Fam Pract 1994; 39:71–75.

PATIENT 46

A 62-year-old man with thickened skin

A 62-year-old man noted painless hardening of the skin over the back and neck of 12 months' duration. Range of motion of the shoulders and neck became limited. He felt generally well and denied symptoms of Raynaud's phenomenon, dysphagia, or dyspnea. There was no history of antecedent illness, or diabetes mellitus.

Physical Examination: Temperature 98.2°, heart rate 80, respiratory rate 18, blood pressure 160/70. Skin: woody induration of skin over the back extending to the neck, face and anterior shoulders, with sparing of the digits. HEENT: normal. Neck: limited extension and rotation. Lungs: clear. Heart: normal. Abdomen: normal. Musculoskeletal: normal. Neurologic: normal. Extremities: no clubbing, cyanosis or edema.

Laboratory Findings: WBC 5,000/μL; Hct 43%; platelets 200,000/μL. Absolute eosinophil count: 200/μL. Westergren ESR: 5 mm/hr. Serum chemistries: normal. Nailfold capillary microscopy: normal. ANA: negative. Scl-70 antibody: negative. Serum protein electrophoresis: small monoclonal protein band in gamma fraction measuring 0.25 g/dL. Immunoelectrophoresis: IgG kappa paraprotein. Skin biopsy: markedly thickened dermis with mucin deposits between and among collagen bundles (see Figure).

Question: What is the diagnosis?

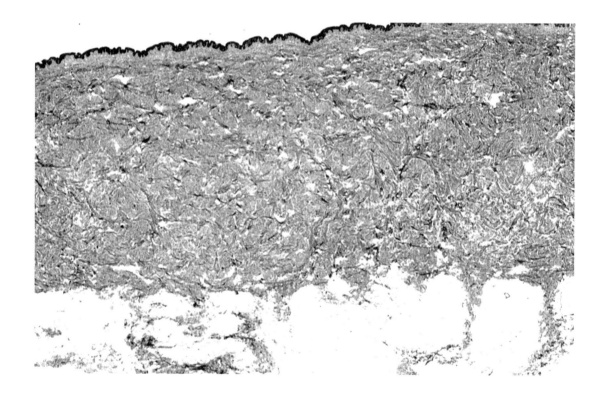

Diagnosis: Scleredema adultorum associated with IgG-kappa paraproteinemia.

Discussion: Scleredema (Buschke's disease) is a rare cutaneous mucinosis characterized clinically by non-pitting induration of the skin. The dermis of the neck, head, and upper trunk usually is involved, while the distal extremities are spared. The absence of acrosclerosis and Raynaud's phenomenon, together with the lack of scleroderma-specific autoantibodies or abnormal nailfold capillary morphology, serve to distinguish scleredema and other cutaneous mucinoses, e.g., scleromyxedema, from systemic sclerosis (scleroderma). The skin has a woody, non-pitting indurated quality, as opposed to the taut, hidebound skin of scleroderma. Eosinophilic fasciitis also should be considered, but it has a predilection for the extremities and is accompanied by blood eosinophilia. Histologically, it may be associated with mucin deposition but is distinguishable by the presence of fasciitis.

Scleredema may have an acute onset after an upper respiratory tract infection (often streptococcal) and in such cases is usually self-limited. Scleredema is also associated with severe diabetes mellitus, in which case it may run a protracted course.

Recently there have been a number of reports of scleredema occurring in association with monoclonal gammopathy. In the majority of cases, an IgG-kappa paraprotein has been detected. In contrast, patients with scleromyxedema (papular mucinosis or lichen myxedematosus) nearly always have a paraprotein, most often of the IgG-lambda type.

Any patient with scleredema should be screened for diabetes mellitus as well as monoclonal gammopathy. Rare cases of scleredema evolving to multiple myeloma have been described, so if a paraprotein is detected further testing should include tests for urine Bence Jones protein, skeletal survey, and bone marrow biopsy.

There is no effective treatment for scleredema, yet many cases resolve spontaneously. Cases associated with multiple myeloma may respond to chemotherapy for multiple myeloma.

In the present patient, a search for multiple myeloma was negative, and no treatment was undertaken. Partial improvement occurred spontaneously.

Clinical Pearls

1. Scleredema is a rare cutaneous mucinosis characterized clinically by non-pitting induration of the skin.

2. Scleredema is distinguishable from scleroderma clinically by the absence of Raynaud's phenomenon and acrosclerosis, negative ANA, normal nailfold capillary morphology, and histologically by the presence of dermal mucin.

3. Scleredema associated with acute respiratory tract infection is usually self-limited, whereas scleredema associated with severe diabetes mellitus is often longstanding.

4. Scleredema may coexist with monoclonal gammopathy, which may rarely evolve to multiple myeloma.

5. IgG-kappa paraproteins are most commonly associated with scleredema; in contrast, patients with paraproteinemia and another cutaneous mucinosis, scleromyxedema, usually exhibit IgG-lambda.

REFERENCES

1. Kovary PM, Vakilzadeh F, Macher E, Zaun H et al. Monoclonal gammopathy in scleredema. Observations in three cases. Arch Dermatol 1981; 117:536–539.
2. McFadden N, Ree K, Soyland E, Larsen TE. Scleredema adultorum associated with a monoclonal gammopathy and generalized hyperpigmentation. Arch Dermatol 1987; 123:629–632.
3. Oikarinen A, Ala-Kokko L, Palatsi R, Peltonen L, Uitto J. Scleredema and paraproteinemia. Enhanced collagen production and elevated type I procollagen messenger RNA level in fibroblasts grown from cultures from the fibrotic skin of a patient. Arch Dermatol 1987; 123:226–229.
4. Hodak E, Tamir R, David M, Hart M et al. Scleredema adultorum associated with IgG-kappa multiple myeloma—a case report and review of the literature. Clin Exp Dermatol 1988; 13:271–274.
5. Sansom JE, Sheehan AL, Kennedy CT, Delaney TJ. A fatal case of scleredema of Buschke. Br J Dermatol 1994; 130:669–670.

PATIENT 47

A 33-year-old woman with a cold foot

A 33-year-old woman had a 1-day history of a cold right foot accompanied by pallor and paresthesias. She denied similar changes in the left foot or hands, although she had a 10-year history of episodic, triphasic color changes of the fingers and toes induced by cold exposure and complicated by digital ulcerations and calcinosis. She also had a long history of dysphagia and gastroesophageal reflux, "broken blood vessels" on the face, and hypertension. At the onset of the present illness she was taking nifedipine, enalapril, and omeprazole.

Physical Examination: Temperature 99.9°; heart rate 128; respiratory rate 18; blood pressure 100/60. Skin: telangiectasias over face and hands; sclerodactyly with healed digital pitted scars. HEENT: circumoral skin furrowing with decreased oral aperture. Chest: normal. Cardiac: normal. Neurologic: normal. Musculoskeletal: normal. Extremities: cold, pale right foot with no palpable pulse over the dorsalis pedis or posterior tibialis artery.

Laboratory Findings: WBC: 14,000/μL with 73% neutrophils, 17% lymphocytes, 10% monocytes. Hct 43.8%; platelets 362,000/μL; ESR 4 mm/hr. Serum chemistries: normal. Urinalysis: normal. Chest radiograph: normal. Echocardiogram: normal. Antiphospholipid antibody and lupus anticoagulant: negative. PT and PTT: normal. Cryoglobulins: negative. ANA: positive, 1:320 centromere pattern. Arteriogram: see below.

Question: What is the diagnosis and treatment?

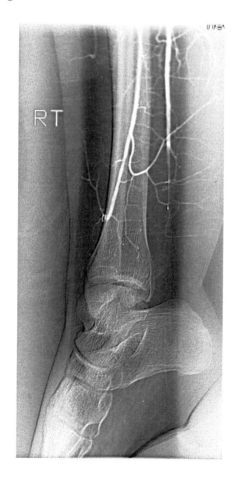

Diagnosis: CREST syndrome with large vessel occlusive disease.

Discussion: Systemic sclerosis (SSc, scleroderma) is classified by the extent of cutaneous involvement and the presence or absence of features of other connective tissue diseases, e.g., systemic lupus erythematosus, polymyositis, and dermatomyositis. In this classification, scleroderma exists as diffuse cutaneous SSc, limited cutaneous SSc, or an overlap syndrome. Patients with limited cutaneous SSc usually have taut skin on the fingers (sclerodactyly) and face and sometimes on the hand and forearm. Many patients with limited cutaneous SSc have Raynaud's phenomenon as the presenting symptom and develop calcinosis, esophageal dysmotility, sclerodactyly, and telangiectasia over the course of many years. This constellation of signs and symptoms is known by the acronym CREST. Approximately 50% of CREST syndrome patients have anticentromere antibodies (ACA).

Obliterative microvascular disease and vasospastic phenomena are hallmarks of SSc, but large vessel occlusive disease is reported infrequently. It would appear, however, that macrovascular disease is more prevalent among SSc patients than in control populations. Large vessel disease may present, as in the present case, with acute pallor and pain due to arterial occlusion, or as intermittent claudication, angina and transient ischemic attacks. Coexisting hypertension, diabetes or hypercholesterolemia may play a role in some cases. Antiphospholipid antibodies, or the lupus anticoagulant, may contribute to large and medium-sized vascular occlusion in some SSc patients. In other cases, such as the present patient, neither atherosclerosis nor antiphospholipid antibodies are detectable. Tests for the lupus anticoagulant and antiphospholipid antibodies were negative, and there was no arteriographic evidence of atherosclerosis. The arteriogram revealed normal vascular anatomy to the level of the right calf, at which point the anterior tibial artery was found to be occluded; the peritoneal and posterior tibial arteries were occluded at the level of the ankle, without arteriographic evidence of atherosclerosis or vasculitis (see Figure).

Medical management of ischemic episodes is often difficult and ineffective. Digital ischemia may respond to vasodilator therapy including calcium-channel blockers, topical nitroglycerin, and chemical sympathectomy. Low-dose aspirin may inhibit platelet aggregation, and pentoxifylline may increase red blood cell flow. Surgical debridement or amputation is sometimes required.

Thrombolytic agents have been shown to improve symptoms and skin blood flow in SSc patients with digital ischemia, but there is little reported experience with thrombolytic therapy for large vessel occlusive disease in SSc patients. In the present case, a microcatheter was advanced into the posterior tibial artery to the level of the occlusion and a bolus of urokinase was given, followed by continuous infusion of urokinase and heparin. Within 24 hours, the foot was warm and the pulses were palpable. Repeat angiography demonstrated a patent posterior tibial artery and plantar arcades reconstituting the distal dorsalis pedis artery. The patient was placed on long-term coumadin therapy.

Clinical Pearls

1. Systemic sclerosis (SSc, scleroderma) is classified by the extent of skin involvement as limited cutaneous or diffuse cutaneous SSc or as an overlap variant with features of systemic lupus erythematosus or poly/dermatomyositis.

2. The limited cutaneous variant of SSc is also known as the CREST syndrome.

3. Approximately 50% of patients with limited cutaneous SSc have the specific anticentromere antibody.

4. Large vessel occlusive disease may occur in SSc patients, particularly those with the CREST variant.

5. Factors contributing to large vessel occlusive disease in some SSc patients include hypertension, atherosclerosis, and antiphospholipid antibodies.

6. Ischemia from large vessel occlusive disease can be improved by thrombolytic therapy.

REFERENCES

1. Shapiro LS. Large vessel arterial thrombosis in systemic sclerosis associated with antiphospholipid antibodies. J Rheumatol 1990; 17:685–688.
2. Klimuik PS, Kay EA, Illingworth KJ, Gush RJ, Taylor LJ, Baker RD, Perkins C, Jayson MIV. A double blind placebo controlled trial of recombinant tissue plasminogen activator in the treatment of digital ischemia in systemic sclerosis. J Rheumatol 1992; 19:716–720.
3. Youssef P, Englert H, Bertouch J. Large vessel occlusive disease associated with CREST syndrome and scleroderma. Ann Rheum Dis 1993; 52:464–466.
4. Veale DJ, Collidge TA, Belch JJF. Increased prevalence of symptomatic macrovascular disease in systemic sclerosis. Ann Rheum Dis 1995; 54:853–855.

PATIENT 48

An 18-year-old boy with left hip pain and anemia

An 18-year-old boy had a 6-month history of left hip pain without antecedent trauma, rash, fever, back pain, gastrointestinal or genitourinary symptoms. This was followed by pain and stiffness affecting the left knee and wrist. There was a remote history of trauma with intermittent pain and swelling of the left knee from a motor vehicle accident. The arthritis had been treated with NSAIDs with only partial improvement.

Physical Examination: Temperature 98.6°; pulse 80; respirations 16; blood pressure 110/70. Skin: normal. HEENT: normal. Chest: clear. Heart: normal. Abdomen: normal. Neurologic: normal. Musculoskeletal: pain and limited range of motion of left hip, knee and wrist; Shöber index: 10cm→15cm.

Laboratory Findings: WBC 12,500/μL; Hct 37.3%; platelets 403,000/μL; MCV 79.5 (80–94); ESR 43 mm/hr; RF and ANA negative; HLA-B27 negative; iron (Fe) 2 μg/dL (35–140); total iron binding capacity (TIBC) 187 μg/dL (245–400); % saturation Fe/TIBC 1% (13–45); serum chemistries normal; urinalysis normal. Sacroiliac radiographs: normal. Hip radiographs: marked loss of left hip joint space (see Figure) with normal right hip.

Question: What procedure led to the correct diagnosis?

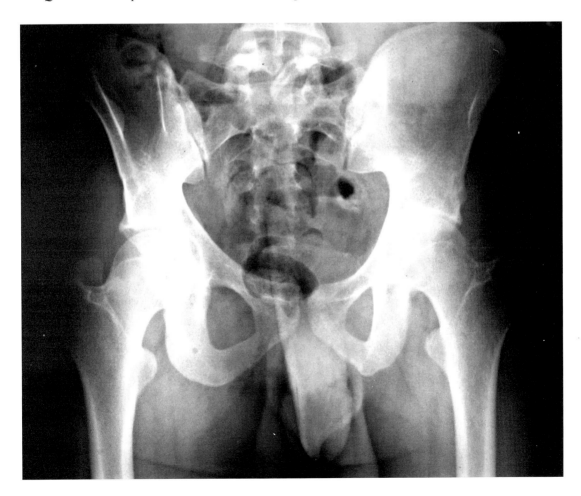

Answer: Gastrointestinal endoscopy; Crohn's disease with enteropathic arthropathy.

Discussion: Arthritis may be a significant extraintestinal manifestation of a number of bowel diseases. Enteropathic arthritis occurs in the following settings: (1) postdysenteric reactive arthritis (Reiter's syndrome); (2) inflammatory bowel disease (ulcerative colitis or Crohn's disease); (3) other conditions such as bowel-bypass syndrome, Whipple's disease, and celiac disease.

Two major types of arthritis may be seen in patients with inflammatory bowel disease (IBD): a peripheral arthritis that is usually asymmetric and oligoarticular, or an axial arthritis involving the sacroiliac, spine, and hip joints. In most cases the intestinal symptoms antedate the arthritis, but occasionally joint disease occurs first.

Peripheral arthritis occurs in up to 20% of IBD patients, with a higher prevalence in Crohn's disease than in ulcerative colitis. There is a predilection for large, lower extremity joints (hips, knees, ankles). Although it is usually nonerosive, destructive joint disease of the hips has been described. As in any synovial disease process, the joint space narrowing occurs as a symmetric process within an individual joint, e.g., hip joint (see Figure). Usually the arthritis is transient, occurring during flares of the bowel disease. In some cases of ulcerative colitis the peripheral arthritis has been cured following total colectomy.

Axial skeletal involvement with sacroiliitis and spondylitis may be seen in either Crohn's disease or ulcerative colitis. Asymptomatic sacroiliitis is present in up to one-third of IBD patients if documented by sensitive techniques such as computed tomography. The onset and course of axial arthritis is independent of the bowel disease, and bowel surgery does not alter its course. The axial arthritis that accompanies IBD is associated with the presence of HLA-B27.

Consider IBD in any patient presenting with a seronegative peripheral or axial arthritis. The presence of occult fecal blood or iron-deficiency anemia should prompt a thorough radiographic or endoscopic evaluation of the gut. Concurrent use of NSAIDs may complicate the picture, since NSAIDs may cause gastrointestinal bleeding and iron deficiency. Other extraintestinal clues of IBD include erythema nodosum, enthesitis, anterior uveitis, aphthous stomatitis, pyoderma gangrenosum, and thrombophlebitis.

In the present case, gastrointestinal endoscopy revealed mild distal esophagitis, superficial erosion of the transverse colon, a multilobulated mass in the cecum measuring 4 cm × 8 cm, and a nodular appearance to the ileum. Surgical biopsy of the cecal mass and ileum revealed submucosal granulomas containing giant cells and chronic inflammation consistent with Crohn's disease. The wrist and knee arthritis improved with sulfasalazine, but chronic hip pain persisted.

Clinical Pearls

1. Enteropathic arthritis occurs as an extraintestinal manifestation of postdysenteric reactive arthritis (Reiter's syndrome), inflammatory bowel disease (IBD), or other conditions such as bowel-bypass syndrome, Whipple's disease or celiac disease.

2. Arthritis may present before, after, or simultaneous with the onset of intestinal symptoms.

3. The prevalence of enteropathic arthritis is higher among Crohn's disease patients than among ulcerative colitis patients.

4. Two major types of arthritis are seen in patients with IBD: (1) a peripheral arthritis that is asymmetric, oligoarticular, predominantly lower extremity that tends to wax and wane with activity of the bowel disease; and (2) an axial arthritis involving the sacroiliac, spine and hip joints associated with HLA B-27, that runs a course independent of the bowel disease.

5. Asymptomatic sacroiliitis is detectable in up to one-third of IBD patients using computed tomography.

6. An erosive monoarthritis, usually of the hip, occurs in some patients with IBD.

REFERENCES

1. Passo MH, Fitzgerald JF, Brant KD. Arthritis associated with inflammatory bowel disease in children. Relationship of joint disease to activity and severity of bowel lesion. Dig Dis Sci 1986;31:492–497.
2. Petty RE, Malleson P. Spondyloarthropathies of childhood. Pediatr Clin North Am 1986;33:1079–1096.
3. Gravallese EM, Kantrowitz FG. Arthritic manifestations of inflammatory bowel disease. Am J Gastroenterol 1988;83:703–709.
4. McEniff N, Eustace S, McCarthy C, et al. Asymptomatic sacroiliitis in inflammatory bowel disease. Assessment by computed tomography. Clin Imaging 1995;19:258–262.

PATIENT 49

A 26-year-old woman with wrist arthritis and splenomegaly

A 26-year-old sexually active woman presented with acute synovitis of the wrists. She gave a history of chills and night sweats but denied fever, rash, dysuria, and vaginal discharge.

Physical examination: Temperature 99.3°, heart rate 100, respirations 16, blood pressure 110/70. Skin: no rash. HEENT: normal. Chest: clear. Heart: normal. Abdomen: spleen palpable three finger-breadths below left costal margin. Genitourinary: normal. Neurologic: normal. Musculoskeletal: synovitis and decreased motion of wrists with severe pain over distal radius and ulna bilaterally.

Laboratory findings: WBC 270,000/μL with 80% neutrophils, 10% lymphocytes, 10% monocytes; Hct 31%; platelets 110,000/μL; serum chemistries normal. ESR 80 mm/hr; RF and ANA negative; synovial fluid WBC 10,600/μL with 73% neutrophils, 4% lymphocytes and 23% monocytes; blood, vaginal and synovial fluid cultures negative; wrist radiographs normal. Bone scan: symmetric polyarticular uptake (see below). MRI: abnormal signal intensity involving the marrow.

Question: What is the cause of this patient's musculoskeletal pain?

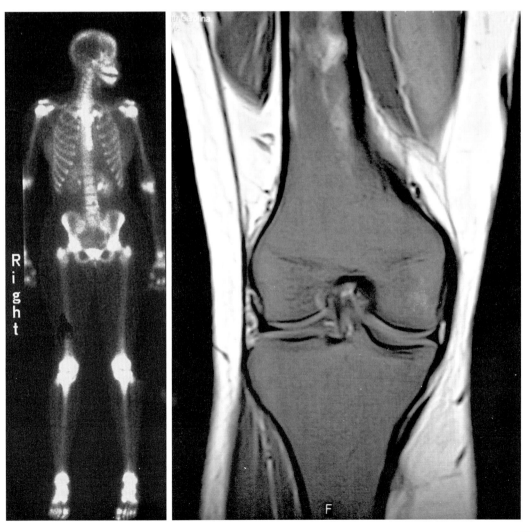

Diagnosis: Chronic myelogenous leukemia.

Discussion: The differential diagnosis of acute monoarthritis or polyarthritis is extensive. Bacterial causes, particularly *Neisseria gonorrhoeae* in sexually active patients, must be sought and, if found, treated with appropriate antibiotics and joint aspiration. Once bacterial arthritis has been excluded, other causes to be considered include crystal-induced arthropathy, rheumatic fever, rheumatoid arthritis, autoimmune connective tissue diseases, seronegative spondyloarthropathy, and various systemic diseases presenting as arthritis.

Leukemia is an uncommon cause of arthritis. Childhood leukemias are complicated by arthritis more frequently than are adult leukemias, and leukemic arthritis occurs more commonly in acute than in chronic leukemia. In nearly one-half of reported cases, joint symptoms preceded recognition of leukemia by a mean of 18 months. In other cases, arthritis occurred simultaneously with the diagnosis of leukemia, or following the diagnosis of leukemia.

Leukemic arthritis may arise from infiltration of leukemic cells into synovium, hemorrhage into the joint from thrombocytopenia, and synovial reaction to periosteal or capsular infiltration. Leukemic blast cells may be present in synovial fluid or synovial tissue. Identification of such cells may be enhanced by indirect immunofluorescent techniques employing monoclonal antibodies against leukemia-associated antigens. Complications of leukemia and its treatment, each of which may present as arthritis, include sepsis, gout, and drug toxicity (especially interferon).

Leukemic arthritis is usually asymmetric and oligoarticular but may be symmetric and polyarticular. Large joints such as knees, ankles, wrists, elbows, shoulders, and hips may be involved. Pain is often severe and out of proportion to the degree of inflammation. Careful examination may disclose that the pain arises more from bone than from joint, especially in childhood leukemia, where metaphyseal radiolucent bands are evident on radiographs in nearly 90% of cases, as compared with fewer than 10% of adult patients.

Treatment with NSAIDs may yield partial benefit, but definitive treatment involves therapy for the leukemia. In many cases the arthritis resolves with hematologic remission, only to reappear during relapse of the leukemia.

In the present case, bone marrow biopsy confirmed the presence of Philadelphia chromosome-positive CML. Treatment of the leukemia was associated with complete resolution of arthritis.

Clinical Pearls

1. Consider leukemia in the differential diagnosis of acute or chronic arthritis.
2. Leukemic arthritis is more common in children than in adults, and more common in acute leukemia than in chronic leukemia.
3. Arthritis may antedate the diagnosis of leukemia, sometimes by months.
4. Metaphyseal radiolucent bands are seen commonly in childhood leukemias but rarely in adult leukemias.
5. Synovial fluid immunocytology may confirm the diagnosis of leukemic arthritis.

REFERENCES

1. Fam AG, Voorneveld C, Robinson JB, et al. Synovial fluid immunocytology in the diagnosis of leukemic synovitis. J Rheumatol 1991;18:293–296.
2. Wandl UB, Nagel-Hiemke M, May D, et al. Lupus-like autoimmune disease induced by interferon therapy for myeloproliferative disorders. Clin Immunol Immunopathol 1992;65:70–74.
3. Evans TI, Nercessian BM, Sanders KM. Leukemic arthritis. Semin Arthritis Rheum 1994;24:48–56.

PATIENT 50

A 50-year-old tennis player with acute calf pain

A 50-year-old man felt a sudden, painful tearing sensation in the calf during the first game of a tennis match. The pain was worse when the foot was plantar-flexed, then suddenly dorsiflexed. There was immediate swelling of the calf, and he could not continue playing tennis. One day later the lower leg and foot appeared bruised. Pain and swelling persisted for weeks, and he sought medical attention.

Physical Examination: Vital signs: normal. General examination: normal. Extremities: full range of motion of knees and ankles; 2 cm asymmetry of calf circumference, right greater than left; tender to palpation at musculotendinous junction of right medial gastrocnemius muscle.

Laboratory Findings: CBC, coagulation tests, serum chemistries: normal. MRI of legs: see Figure.

Question: What is the cause of this tennis player's leg pain?

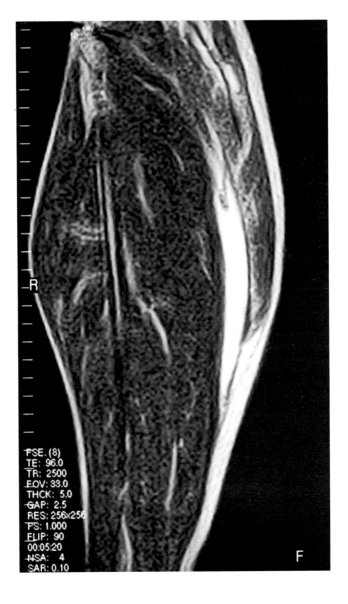

Diagnosis: Rupture of the plantaris muscle, or "tennis leg."

Discussion: Strains or tears of the plantaris muscle or of the medial head of the gastrocnemius muscle, sometimes referred to as "tennis leg," are seen in tennis players older than 40 years. Similar injuries in middle-aged persons engaged in other athletic endeavors, such as skiing or stair-stepping exercises have been observed. Typically, the individual experiences a sudden, painful tearing sensation in the calf muscle with immediate disability and swelling, followed by ecchymosis progressing down the leg into the ankle and foot. Palpation may reveal minimal swelling in a first-degree strain, ranging to a defect in the medial head of the gastrocnemius at the musculotendinous juncture in a severe strain. Conventional radiography and bone scanning have little value in the diagnosis of soft tissue injury. Ultrasonography and MRI scanning may demonstrate fluid collections and muscle tears. As shown in the Figure, an MRI scan reveals an intramuscular hematoma between the soleus muscle and the medial head of the gastrocnemius. The plantaris muscle, which is absent in 7 to 10% of the population, ranges from 7 to 13 cm long, with the myotendinous junction occurring at the level of the origin of the soleus muscle in the proximal portion of the lower leg.

Other causes of acute calf pain to be considered include dissection or rupture of a popliteal cyst; rupture of the Achilles tendon; and deep vein thrombosis. The latter is more likely to occur in a sedentary individual, whereas all of the former conditions typically occur during exercise. Rupture or dissection of a popliteal cyst is usually antedated by knee swelling. Rupture of the Achilles tendon usually occurs 1 to 2 inches proximal to the distal attachment of the tendon on the calcaneus. A characteristic "pop" sensation is felt, with an inability to stand on tiptoes. A positive Thompson test (failure of plantar flexion with passive compression of the gastrocnemius on the affected side) is present with rupture of the Achilles tendon but not with strain or tear of the medial head of the gastrocnemius.

Acute care of plantaris or gastrocnemius muscle strain consists of ice, restricted activity, gentle stretching exercises, heel lifts, and a progressive strengthening program. Immobilization and non-weight-bearing may be necessary in more severe cases to allow complete healing of the muscle.

In the present case, complete recovery occurred following a period of restricted activity.

Clinical Pearls

1. "Tennis leg" refers to strains or tears of the plantaris muscle or of the medial head of the gastrocnemius, usually occurring in tennis players over the age of 40, but also occurring in other athletic activities.

2. Consider the diagnosis in the athlete complaining of sudden, painful tearing sensation in the calf muscles with immediate swelling followed by ecchymosis progressing down the leg.

3. The differential diagnosis includes rupture of a popliteal cyst, rupture of the Achilles tendon, or deep vein thrombosis.

4. MR imaging may reveal an intermuscular hematoma between the soleus muscle and the medial head of the gastrocnemius muscle; an associated partial tear of the medial head of the gastrocnemius muscle also may be observed.

REFERENCES

1. Gilbert T, Ansari A. A tennis player with a swollen calf. Hosp Pract 1991;26:209–210,212.
2. Menz MJ, Lucas GL. Magnetic resonance imaging of a rupture of the medial head of the gastrocnemius muscle. A case report. J Bone Joint Surg (Am) 1991;73:1260–1262.
3. O'Neil R. Chapter 7. Foot, ankle and lower leg. In: Anderson MK, Hall SJ (eds). Sports Injury Management. Baltimore, Williams & Wilkins, 1995, pp 248–249.
4. Helms CA, Fritz RC, Garvin GJ. Plantaris muscle injury: evaluation with MR imaging. Radiology 1995;195:201–203.

PATIENT 51

A 19-year-old woman with inflammatory bowel disease and low back pain

A 19-year-old woman presented with a 3-day history of low back pain. At age 12 she had inflammatory bowel disease and symmetric polyarthritis involving the ankles and knees that responded to sulfasalazine, prednisone, and nonsteroidal anti-inflammatory drugs. She required total colectomy, and subsequently an ileoanal pouch was created. Although she had no recurrence of peripheral arthritis, at age 18 she complained of right-sided low back pain. One year later she noted similar pain on the left.

Physical Examination: Temperature 97.2°; pulse 80; respirations 18; blood pressure 94/60. Skin: normal. HEENT: normal. Lungs: clear. Cardiac: normal. Abdomen: nontender. Musculoskeletal: normal peripheral joints; tender to palpation over each sacroiliac joint with normal Schöber index.

Laboratory Findings: WBC 10,300/μL; Hct 41.6%; platelet count 338,000/μL. Urinalysis: normal. Westergren ESR: 5 mm/hr. Hip and sacroiliac radiographs: see Figure.

Question: What is the cause of this patient's back pain?

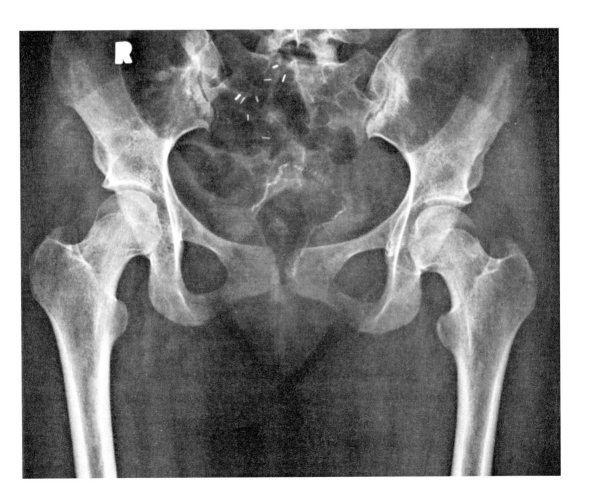

Diagnosis: Sacroiliitis associated with inflammatory bowel disease.

Discussion: Inflammatory bowel disease may be complicated by arthritis involving peripheral joints or axial skeletal joints. In both Crohn's disease and ulcerative colitis, arthritis may antedate the onset of bowel symptoms. Arthritis may also occur simultaneously with bowel symptoms, as did the peripheral arthritis in the present patient; or it may appear years later, as the present patient experienced with her sacroiliitis.

Peripheral arthritis associated with inflammatory bowel disease most often is oligoarticular and asymmetric, with a predilection for the lower extremities. In ulcerative colitis, attacks of arthritis usually occur in temporal relation to flares of colitis. Although peripheral arthritis is cured by total colectomy in most patients, some may have their first episode of arthritis after placement of an ileoanal pouch.

Unlike peripheral arthritis, axial arthritis runs a course independent of the bowel disease. Clinically apparent sacroiliitis occurs in up to 20% of patients, but asymptomatic sacroiliitis has been identified in 32% of patients with inflammatory bowel disease examined by computed tomography. Spondylitis is less prevalent. Patients complain of back pain that is inflammatory in nature (insidious onset, morning stiffness, improvement with exercise). They may have buttock, chest, cervical, or thoracic pain. Sacroiliac pain can be distinguished from hip pain by careful physical examination and radiographic studies.

Radiographic findings of sacroiliitis include blurring of the joint margin, subchondral sclerosis, pseudo-widening or erosions, and partial or complete ankylosis. Although classically the sacroiliitis in patients with inflammatory bowel disease is like that of ankylosing spondylitis, i.e., bilateral and symmetric, the present patient illustrates that early in the course it may be bilateral and asymmetric (see Figure). Unilateral sacroiliitis is a red flag for infection, but also may occur in Reiter syndrome and psoriatic spondylitis.

Treatment of arthritis associated with inflammatory bowel disease entails the use of nonsteroidal anti-inflammatory drugs and intra-articular corticosteroids. Systemic steroids and other agents for control of bowel symptoms may improve the peripheral arthritis. Sulfasalazine may improve both the gut and the joint disease, including axial skeletal joints.

The present patient had inflammatory bowel disease with both peripheral arthritis and sacroiliac arthritis. Radiographs revealed erosions and sclerosis involving the lower two-thirds of the sacroiliac joints. Initially the sclerosis was bilateral and asymmetric, but later was bilateral and symmetric. The patient was treated with low-dose steroids, NSAIDs, and sulfasalazine. The peripheral arthritis waxed and waned in accord with the degree of "pouchitis," but sacroiliitis persisted even when the bowel disease appeared to be inactive.

Clinical Pearls

1. Peripheral arthritis associated with inflammatory bowel disease runs a course that parallels the activity of the bowel disease.

2. In ulcerative colitis, peripheral arthritis may be cured by total colectomy, although arthritis may first occur after placement of an ileoanal pouch.

3. Axial arthritis runs a course independent of the bowel disease activity.

4. Sacroiliitis is a frequent extraintestinal manifestation of inflammatory bowel disease and may occur in 30% of asymptomatic patients.

5. The sacroiliitis of inflammatory bowel disease is typically bilateral and symmetric, but early cases may be bilateral and asymmetric.

REFERENCES

1. Resnick D, Niwayama G. Ankylosing spondylitis. In: Resnick D, Niwayama G (eds). Diagnosis of Bone and Joint Disorders, 2d ed. Philadelphia, WB Saunders, 1988, pp 1103–1170.
2. Ferraz MB, Tugwell P, Goldsmith CH, Atra E: Meta-analysis of sulfasalazine in ankylosing spondylitis. J Rheumatol 1990;17:1482–1486.
3. Axon JM, Hawley PR, Huskisson EC: Ileal pouch arthritis. Br J Rheumatol 1993;32:586–588.
4. McEniff N, Eustace S, McCarthy C, et al: Asymptomatic sacroiliitis in inflammatory bowel disease. Assessment by computed tomography. Clin Imaging 1995;19:258–262.

PATIENT 52

A 47-year-old woman with a pulmonary-renal syndrome

A 47-year-old woman had a 3-month history of malaise, arthralgia, low-grade fever, and cough. The cough was accompanied by dyspnea and hemoptysis. She had a long history of sinusitis but denied headache or bloody nasal discharge.

Physical Examination: Temperature 100.2°; heart rate 100, regular; respirations 18; blood pressure 110/70. General: ill appearance. Skin: no rash. HEENT: normal. Neck: normal. Chest: bibasilar crackles. Cardiac: normal. Abdomen: normal. Neurologic: normal. Extremities: normal.

Laboratory Findings: WBC 8900/μL; Hct 30.4%; platelet count 375,000/μL; BUN 35 mg/dL; creatinine 2.3 mg/dL. Urinalysis: 1+ protein, 25 WBC/hpf, > 1000 RBC/hpf; ESR 110 mm/hr; serum C3 and C4 normal; ANCA: positive with perinuclear pattern (antimyeloperoxidase positive). Chest radiograph: bilateral patchy infiltrates; sinus CT scan: normal. Renal biopsy: focal, segmental, pauci-immune glomerulonephritis; lung biopsy: small vessel vasculitis with pulmonary hemorrhage, mild interstitial fibrosis, and no granulomata.

Question: What is the diagnosis?

Diagnosis: Microscopic polyangiitis (MPA).

Discussion: Systemic vasculitis may present as a pulmonary-renal syndrome characterized by hemoptysis and rapidly progressive glomerulonephritis. The major rheumatic diseases capable of producing a pulmonary-renal syndrome are systemic lupus erythematosus (SLE), Goodpasture syndrome, Wegener granulomatosis, and microscopic polyangiitis (MPA). Patients with pulmonary-renal syndrome related to SLE have characteristic skin lesions, serologic abnormalities (low serum complement levels and positive anti-DNA antibodies), and immune complex-mediated glomerulonephritis. Goodpasture syndrome is defined by the presence of antibodies to glomerular basement membrane in the serum, lung, or renal tissue. In contrast, Wegener granulomatosis and MPA lack significant renal immunopathology; i.e., the glomerulonephritis is "pauci-immune." Wegener granulomatosis is distinguished by granulomatous vasculitis of the respiratory tract, usually in association with glomerulonephritis and antineutrophil cytoplasmic antibody directed against proteinase-3 (c-ANCA). Although the ANCA is also positive in MPA, such patients lack granulomatous airway disease and usually (50–80%) have a perinuclear antineutrophil cytoplasmic staining pattern (p-ANCA) representing antibodies to myeloperoxidase.

MPA must also be distinguished from classic polyarteritis nodosa (PAN). Histologic differentiation may not always be possible, but clinical, serologic, and radiographic studies support the distinction. Unlike PAN, patients with MPA frequently have lung involvement and p-ANCA, negative hepatitis virus serologies, and no arteriographic evidence of microaneurysms. Therapy differs for MPA and PAN. PAN usually responds to steroids and immunosuppressive drugs, or, in the case of hepatitis-associated PAN, to antiviral agents and plasmapheresis. Prognosis is good and relapses are rare. MPA, on the other hand, may be complicated by fatal pulmonary hemorrhage or chronic renal failure, and relapses are common. Severe MPA is treated with intravenous pulse methylprednisolone, oral or pulse cyclophosphamide, and plasmapheresis if there is pulmonary hemorrhage. High-dose intravenous immunoglobulin (IgG) therapy may produce clinical improvement and a fall in ANCA titer.

The present patient's pulmonary-renal syndrome with pauci-immune glomerulonephritis, p-ANCA, and absence of granulomatous vasculitis of the respiratory tract was consistent with microscopic polyangiitis (MPA). She was treated with high-dose corticosteroids, cyclophosphamide, plasmapheresis, and intravenous IgG. Her course was complicated by hemorrhagic cystitis and leukopenia. She died from fungal pneumonia; at autopsy there was evidence of active MPA.

Clinical Pearls

1. Systemic vasculitis causing a pulmonary-renal syndrome may be a feature of systemic lupus erythematosus, Goodpasture syndrome, Wegener granulomatosis, or microscopic polyangiitis (MPA).

2. MPA is a small-vessel vasculitis (capillaries, venules, arterioles) with nongranulomatous pauci-immune glomerulonephritis.

3. MPA is distinguished from classic polyarteritis nodosa (PAN) on clinical, serologic, and arteriographic grounds.

4. Most patients (50–80%) with MPA have antineutrophil cytoplasmic antibodies with a perinuclear staining pattern (p-ANCA) that represent antibodies to myeloperoxidase.

5. Treatment of MPA consists of pulse methylprednisolone, cyclophosphamide, and in some cases plasmapheresis and intravenous IgG.

REFERENCES

1. Geffriaud-Ricouard C, Noel LH, Chareau D, et al. Clinical spectrum associated with ANCA of defined antigen specificities in 98 selected patients. Clin Nephrol 1993;39:125–136.
2. Jennette C, Falk R, Andrassy K, et al. Nomenclature of systemic vasculitides: proposal of an international consensus conference. Arthritis Rheum 1994;37:187–192.
3. Guillevin L, Lhote F. Distinguishing polyarteritis nodosa from microscopic polyangiitis and implications for treatment. Curr Opin Rheumatol 1995;7:20–24.

PATIENT 53

A 57-year-old woman with back and hip pain and an elevated sedimentation rate

A 57-year-old woman developed diffuse low back and hip pain 2 years after undergoing lumpectomy and radiation therapy for breast cancer. The pain was worse with sitting and at night and improved with walking. Although she complained of morning stiffness, there was no joint pain or swelling, shoulder girdle stiffness, weight loss, headache, jaw claudication, or visual disturbances. Her back and hip symptoms had not improved with prednisone, 20 mg/day, but were somewhat improved with ibuprofen.

Physical Examination: Vital signs: normal. Musculoskeletal: no peripheral joint synovitis; back without point tenderness over vertebral bodies. Neurologic: normal lower extremity strength, reflexes, and sensation.

Laboratory Findings: WBC 5500/μL; Hct 32%; Westergren ESR 85 mm/hr; C-reactive protein <0.1 mg/dL; electrolytes, BUN, creatinine, liver function tests normal; calcium 9.8 mg/dL, phosphorus 3.2 mg/dL. Urinalysis: no protein, cells, or casts. Radiographs and MRI scan of the lumbar spine: normal. Serumprotein electrophoresis: (see Figure).

Questions: What is a likely diagnosis? How should the diagnosis be pursued?

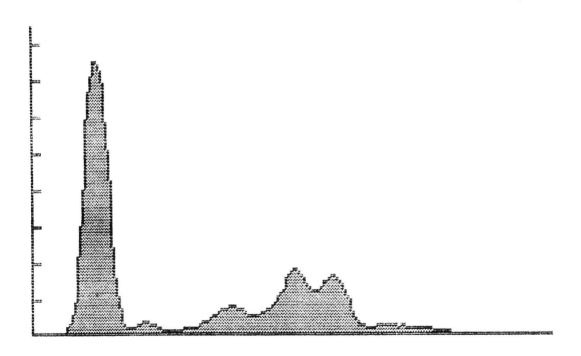

Diagnosis: IgM myeloma.

Discussion: Back and hip pain in an individual over 50 can result from many causes. Spondylosis should be considered and symptoms and signs of nerve root compression (paresthesias, weakness, bladder or bowel dysfunction, reflex abnormalities) sought. Osteoarthritis of the hip joint is characterized by inguinal pain worsened by weight bearing. Muscular back pain often follows an identifiable activity and improves with time and rest.

Back pain as a result of metastatic malignancy is often severe, unremitting, worsened by weight bearing, and worse at night. There is often point tenderness over the spinous process of the involved vertebra. The pedicle is most commonly involved radiographically, but involvement may be isolated to the vertebral body. At times, there is a diffusely radiopaque vertebral body, the so-called ivory vertebral body.

Low back pain may accompany shoulder and pelvic girdle symptoms in polymyalgia rheumatica. Generally there are no physical findings other than tenderness and decreased mobility unless polymyalgia rheumatica is accompanied by temporal arteritis. There is always laboratory evidence of the acute phase response, such as elevated sedimentation rate and C-reactive protein.

Back pain can result from multiple myeloma due to plasma cell infiltration of the vertebral body or pelvis. A plasmacytoma may impinge on the spinal cord and cause pain and neurologic abnormalities. An elevated erythrocyte sedimentation rate can result from activation of the acute phase response or from an elevation of serum immunoglobulin levels. When there is an elevation of the sedimentation rate without an accompanying increase in acute phase proteins, a search for paraproteinemia is warranted.

The present patient was initially treated for polymyalgia rheumatica but did not respond to prednisone. A bone scan, performed because of the history of breast cancer, showed increased activity within two adjacent thoracic vertebral bodies. Urinary protein electrophoresis was normal, but serum protein electrophoresis showed a monoclonal spike in the beta region. The monoclonal protein was an IgM kappa at a concentration of 0.89 g/dL. Serum IgG and IgA levels were diminished at 593 and 60 mg/dL, respectively.

Treatment was initiated with prednisone, 20 mg orally three times daily, and melphalan, 0.15 mg per kilogram orally for 7 days. This therapy was repeated for three cycles every 6 weeks. Currently the patient is free of back pain and anemia.

Clinical Pearls

1. An elevated sedimentation rate without accompanying increases in acute phase proteins, such as C-reactive protein, must prompt an evaluation for a plasma cell dyscrasia, such as multiple myeloma or macroglubulinemia.

2. Metastatic disease to the spine generally causes severe, unremitting back pain.

3. Multiple myeloma may cause back pain when vertebral bone marrow is involved or when a plasmacytoma impinges on the spine or neural structures.

REFERENCES

1. Ucci G, Riccardi A, Luoni R, Ascari E. Presenting features of monoclonal gammopathies: an analysis of 684 newly diagnosed cases. Cooperative Group for the Study and Treatment of Multiple Myeloma. J Intern Med 1993;234:165–173.
2. Talstad I, Haugen HF. The relationship between the erythrocyte sedimentation rate (ESR) and plasma proteins in clinical materials and models. Scan J Clin Lab Invest 1979;39:519–524.
3. Case records of the Massachusetts General Hospital. Weekly clinicopathological exercises. Case 20–1977. N Engl J Med 1977;19;296:1156–1163.

PATIENT 54

A 56-year-old man with scleroderma and a lung lesion

A 56-year-old man was found to have a left upper lobe lesion on a routine chest radiograph. He smoked cigarettes and had an 8-year history of systemic sclerosis, which was complicated by interstitial pulmonary fibrosis, esophageal dysmotility, hypertension, and cardiac arrhythmias requiring a pacemaker. Dyspnea and restrictive lung disease improved with cyclophosphamide treatment, which was discontinued 4 years prior to detection of the lung lesion.

Physical Examination: Temperature 98.6°; heart rate 80, regular; respirations 20; blood pressure 180/86. Skin: sclerodactyly. Nodes: negative. HEENT: normal. Chest: clear. Cardiac: paced rhythm. Abdomen: normal. Neurologic: normal. Genitalia: penile prosthesis. Extremities: 1+ edema.

Laboratory Findings: WBC 7700/μL; Hct 42.9%; platelet count 171,000/μL. Serum chemistries: normal. Urinalysis: normal. ANA: positive, 1:640 with nucleolar pattern. Anti-Scl-70 antibody: positive. Chest radiograph: see Figure.

Question: What is a leading diagnostic possibility?

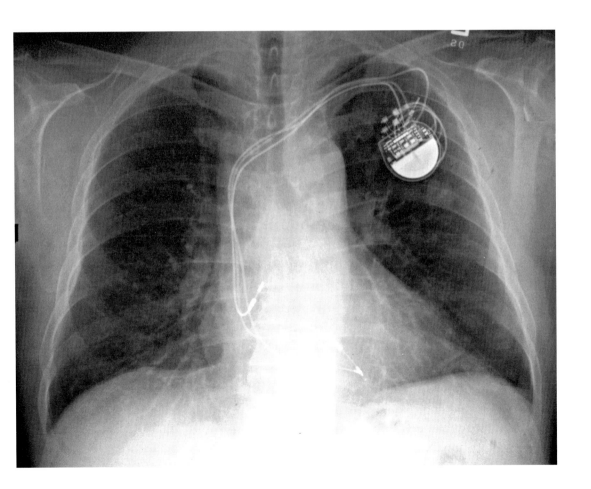

Diagnosis: Carcinoma of the lung.

Discussion: The pulmonary manifestations of systemic sclerosis (scleroderma) include interstitial fibrosis, pulmonary hypertension, pleural disease, aspiration pneumonia, and malignancy. There is an overall twofold increased incidence of cancer among patients with systemic sclerosis, and lung cancer is the most frequent neoplasm reported in association with this disease. One population-based study found the standardized incidence ratio for lung cancer to equal 7.8. The presence of pulmonary fibrosis, as in the present patient, appears to be a risk factor for lung cancer in scleroderma. Various types of lung tumors may occur in scleroderma, including alveolar, bronchiolar, adenocarcinoma, and squamous cell carcinoma. Other neoplasms that may occur more frequently in scleroderma are breast cancer and non-Hodgkin's lymphoma.

As in the present patient, scleroderma usually is present for many years before the detection of malignancy. The increased prevalence of carcinoma at any site of scar tissue is well appreciated and may explain the increased risk of lung cancer in scleroderma. In one study of 680 scleroderma patients, 62% of those with pulmonary malignancy had evidence of lung fibrosis, whereas only 28% of those without malignancy had lung fibrosis. Diffuse fibrosis causes thickening of alveolar walls with subsequent obliteration and generation of small cysts. These cystic spaces undergo epithelial proliferation, and attempts at cellular regeneration in the setting of altered immunity may predispose to the development of malignancy.

Anti-Scl-70 antibodies (anti-DNA topoisomerase I) have been reported to be associated with malignancy, especially lung cancer, in patients with scleroderma. Anti-Scl-70 antibody levels may rise markedly at the time of diagnosis of lung cancer, perhaps due to increased topoisomerase I expression by malignant cells.

In the present case, risk factors for lung cancer included tobacco use, scleroderma with pulmonary fibrosis, anti-Scl-70 antibodies, and a history of immunosuppressive drug treatment. The patient underwent thoracotomy and left upper lobe resection. Two masses measuring 4.5 cm and 3 cm in diameter were found to represent poorly differentiated squamous cell carcinoma with extension to peribronchial nodes.

Clinical Pearls

1. Patients with scleroderma (systemic sclerosis) have an increased incidence of neoplasm compared with population-based control subjects.

2. Lung, breast, and non-Hodgkin's lymphoma occur with increased frequency among patients with scleroderma.

3. Lung cancer in scleroderma patients is associated with the presence of pulmonary fibrosis and antibodies to topoisomerase I (Scl-70).

4. Anti-Scl-70 antibody titers may increase markedly at the time of diagnosis of lung cancer.

REFERENCES

1. Talbott JH, Barrocas M. Carcinoma of the lung in progressive systemic sclerosis: a tabular review of the literature and a detailed report of the roentgenographic changes in two cases. Sem Arthritis Rheum 1980;9:191–217.
2. Roumm AD, Medsger TA Jr. Cancer in systemic sclerosis: an epidemiologic study. Arthritis Rheum 1984;27:S19.
3. Rothfield N, Kurtzman S, Vazques-Abad D, et al. Association of anti-topoisomerase I with cancer. Arthritis Rheum 1992;35:724.
4. Rosenthal AK, McLaughlin JK, Linet MS, Persson I. Scleroderma and malignancy: an epidemiological study. Ann Rheum Dis 1993;52:531–533.
5. Abu-Shakra M, Guillemin F, Lee P. Cancer in systemic sclerosis. Arthritis Rheum 1993;36:460–464.
6. Conaghan PG, Brooks PM. Rheumatic manifestations of malignancy. Curr Opin Rheumatol 1994;6:105–110.
7. Kuwana M, Fujii T, Mimori T, et al. Enhancement of anti-DNA topoisomerase I autoantibody response after lung cancer in patients with systemic sclerosis. Arthritis Rheum 1996;39:686–691.

PATIENT 55

A 16-year-old girl with appendicitis, myalgia, and arthralgias

A 16-year-old girl presented with acute abdominal pain; at laparotomy she was found to have appendicitis and necrotizing arteritis of the vermiform appendix. Her only other complaints were fatigue, myalgias, and arthralgias beginning 2 months prior to the onset of abdominal pain. She had acne but no other skin rash. She denied fever, chills, night sweats, cough, dyspnea, or sinus headaches.

Physical Examination: Temperature 98.2°; heart rate 70; respirations 12; blood pressure 104/78. Skin: facial acne. Nodes: negative. HEENT: normal. Chest: normal. Cardiac: normal. Abdomen: mild tenderness over healing incision; no bruit, mass, or hepatosplenomegaly. Rectal: normal. Genitalia: normal. Neurologic: normal.

Laboratory Findings: WBC 17,500/μL with normal differential; Hct 35.7%; platelet count 365,000/μL; electrolytes, renal indices, and liver function tests normal. RF negative; ANA positive, 1:160 speckled; anti-DNA negative; C3 and C4 normal; hepatitis virus serologies negative; ANCA positive, 1:1280, cytoplasmic pattern; anti-PR3 negative. Urinalysis: 1+ proteinuria, no cells or casts. Sinus CT scan: normal; mesenteric arteriogram: see Figure.

Question: What is the diagnosis?

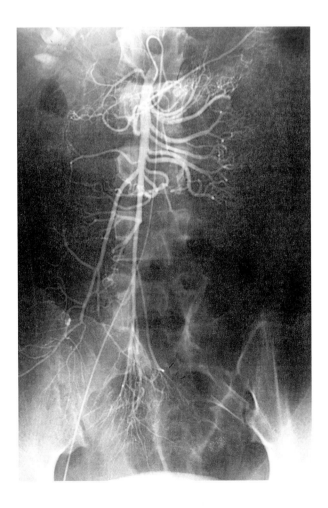

Diagnosis: Systemic polyarteritis nodosa (PAN).

Discussion: Classic PAN is an acute or subacute systemic vasculitis involving medium and small muscular arteries. Necrosis of the vessel wall occurs without granulomas. Frequent clinical manifestations include fever, malaise, peripheral neuropathy, arthralgias, myalgias, and visceral organ involvement. The gastrointestinal tract, kidneys, and heart are often involved. Unlike Wegener granulomatosis and microscopic polyangiitis (MPA), glomerulonephritis and pulmonary involvement are rare, and ANCA is uncommon (< 20%). ANCA, when present, usually has a perinuclear staining pattern (p-ANCA), but lacks the specificity for myeloperoxidase seen in MPA.

The etiology of classic PAN is unknown, but a variable proportion of cases are associated with hepatitis B virus (HBV) infection. Recently, cases of PAN-like vasculitis have been reported in association with human immunodeficiency virus (HIV) infection.

In rare cases, PAN may present as necrotizing vasculitis of the vermiform appendix. Unlike classic PAN, which affects middle-aged males more often than females, patients with necrotizing vasculitis of the vermiform appendix are young and more likely to be female. Although necrotizing vasculitis of the appendix is commonly asymptomatic, some patients do have symptoms and are found to have a systemic vasculitis. Colonic perforation due to ulceration or infarction of the colon secondary to necrotizing mesenteric vasculitis can be fatal in such cases.

Mesenteric angiography may confirm the diagnosis of PAN in cases of necrotizing vasculitis of the vermiform appendix. Histopathologic examination of involved vessels is the preferred method of diagnosis, but when biopsy is not feasible arteriography may be confirmatory. The presence of aneurysms or occlusions of mesenteric and renal vessels, not caused by atherosclerosis, is consistent with PAN. In some cases, large visceral aneurysms may rupture. Percutaneous coil embolization has been reported to be successful in a few such patients. Treatment of PAN entails the use of steroids and/or cytotoxic agents, or antiviral agents and plasma exchange for HBV-related PAN.

In the present patient, necrotizing vasculitis of the vermiform appendix was found at laparotomy, and angiography revealed aneurysms and occlusion of visceral arteries, thus confirming the diagnosis of systemic vasculitis (PAN-type). The patient was treated with high-dose corticosteroids, and all symptoms resolved. ANCA titer decreased and arteriographic abnormalities improved. The patient remained well off corticosteroids.

Clinical Pearls

1. PAN is a systemic necrotizing vasculitis affecting medium and small muscular arteries; sometimes it is associated with HBV or HIV infection.

2. Unlike MPA, classic PAN rarely is complicated by rapidly progressive glomerulonephritis or pulmonary hemorrhage, and the ANCA, if present, is usually nonspecific.

3. PAN may present as necrotizing vasculitis of the vermiform appendix.

4. In some cases, necrotizing vasculitis of the vermiform appendix is isolated to the appendix, but in other cases angiographic evidence of aneurysms and vasculopathy confirms the diagnosis of systemic PAN.

5. Clinical remission is associated with disappearance or regression of aneurysms.

REFERENCES

1. Moyana TN. Necrotizing arteritis of the vermiform appendix. Arch Pathol Lab Med 1988;112:738–741.
2. Darras-Joly C, Lortholary O, Cohen P, et al. Regressing microaneurysms in five cases of hepatitis B virus related to polyarteritis nodosa. J Rheumatol 1995;22:876–880.
3. Libman BS, Quismorio FP Jr, Stimmler MM. Polyarteritis nodosa-like vasculitis in human immunodeficiency virus infection. J Rheumatol 1995;22:351–355.
4. Hachulla E, Bourdon F, Taieb S, et al. Embolization of two bleeding aneurysms with platinum coils in a patient with polyarteritis nodosa. J Rheumatol 1993;20:158–161.
5. Guillevin L, Lhote F. Distinguishing polyarteritis nodosa from microscopic polyangiitis and implications for treatment. Curr Opin Rheumatol 1995;7:20–24.

PATIENT 56

A 54-year-old man with painful thigh muscles

A 54-year-old man with a 5-year history of diabetes mellitus and coronary artery disease developed bilateral thigh pain. Two weeks later the left anterior thigh became indurated and more painful. He had no weakness, but the severity of the pain limited walking. His only medication was glyburide.

Physical Examination: Vital signs: normal. Extremities: induration of the left lateral thigh with exquisite tenderness of both quadriceps muscles.

Laboratory Findings: WBC 13,500/μL with 60% neutrophils, 13% lymphocytes, 7% monocytes; Hct 40%; platelet count 303,000/μL. Electrolytes, BUN, creatinine, and liver function tests: normal. Urinalysis: 100 mg/dL protein, 500 mg/dL glucose. CPK: 109 IU/mL (44–180). Westergren ESR: 92 mm/hr. Biopsy of left lateral quadriceps femoris muscle (see Figure).

Question: What is the diagnosis?

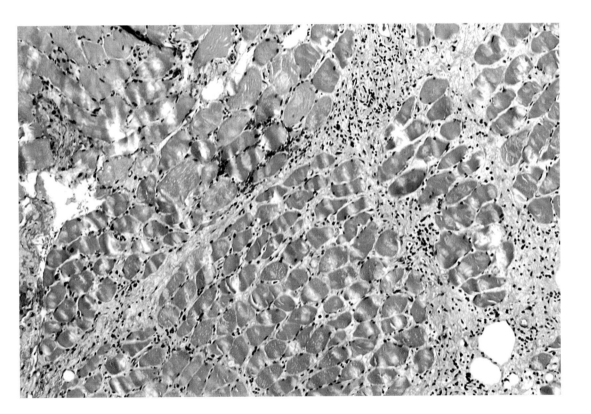

Diagnosis: Diabetic muscle infarction.

Discussion: Subacute, painful, and swollen muscle can result from only a few pathologic processes. Intramuscular hemorrhage from trauma or a coagulation defect can cause this picture, but is easily excluded by history and laboratory testing. Tropical pyomyositis resulting from staphylococcal infection is seen only in the tropics and is the result of spread from a localized skin infection. Inflammatory muscle disease (poly- or dermatomyositis) is characterized by weakness rather than pain, and is associated with proximal more than distal musculature. One unusual form of inflammatory muscle disease is "localized myositis" in which just one muscle or muscle group is involved. The pathologic features are those of idiopathic inflammatory muscle disease: inflammatory cell infiltrate with degeneration and regeneration of muscle fibers. Diabetic muscle infarction is the other entity to be considered in this setting.

Diabetic muscle infarction generally occurs in patients with longstanding, poorly controlled diabetes mellitus. The clinical picture is that of a painful, swollen, and tender thigh, either unilateral or bilateral. Most patients are insulin-dependent, and the first patients to be described had evidence of end-organ involvement, particularly renal disease with proteinuria or uremia. More recent case reports include type II diabetics, but most have atherosclerosis and poor glycemic control. The pathologic findings on biopsy are muscle necrosis and inflammation (see Figure).

Treatment of diabetic muscle infarction includes analgesics and glycemic control, with rehabilitation when pain subsides. Immunosuppression is not beneficial, and corticosteroids may only worsen the situation.

The present patient had been started on steroids initially, as he was believed to have had localized myositis. There was no improvement over a 6-week period, and control of his glucose became quite difficult. Prednisone was stopped, pain control was instituted, and gentle physical therapy was begun. He improved gradually over a 4-month period.

CLINICAL PEARLS

1. Diabetic muscle infarction occurs in the setting of poorly controlled diabetes, most often in patients with evidence of end-organ damage.

2. Patients with diabetic muscle infarction complain of severe unilateral or bilateral thigh pain. Swelling, induration, and erythema of the quadriceps muscle are characteristic.

3. Treatment of diabetic muscle infarction involves analgesics, control of blood glucose, and gentle exercise. Corticosteroids are not helpful and should be avoided.

REFERENCES

1. Barton KL, Palmer BF. Bilateral infarction of the vastus lateralis muscle in a diabetic patient: a case report and review of the literature. J Diabetes Complications 1993;7:221–223.
2. Rocca PV, Alloway JA, Nashel DJ. Diabetic muscular infarction. Semin Arthritis Rheum 1993;22:280–287.
3. Bodner RA, Younger DS, Rosoklija G. Diabetic muscle infarction. Muscle Nerve 1994;17:949–950.
4. Bjornskov EK, Carry MR, Katz FH, et al. Diabetic muscle infarction: a new perspective on pathogenesis and management. Neuromuscul Disord 1995;5:39–45.

PATIENT 57

A 51-year-old patient with scleroderma, abdominal pain, vomiting, and diarrhea

A 51-year-old man had a 1-year history of diffuse cutaneous systemic sclerosis (scleroderma) characterized by Raynaud phenomenon, dysphagia, sclerodactyly and taut truncal skin, restrictive lung disease, and abnormal nailfold capillary morphology. He presented with a 5-day history of nausea, vomiting, diarrhea, abdominal distention, and pain. In the preceding months he had a 7-pound weight loss. There was no history of fever, chills, hematemesis, or hematochezia.

Physical Examination: Temperature 97.8°; heart rate 72; respirations 16; blood pressure 120/70. Skin: pitted digital scars on fingertips, sclerodactyly, and truncal skin sclerosis. HEENT: decreased oral aperture. Chest: dry basilar rales. Heart: normal. Abdomen: mildly tender and distended with diminished bowel sounds. Rectal: no stool. Neurologic: normal. Musculoskeletal: flexion contractures of the fingers; no synovitis.

Laboratory Findings: Hct 35%; WBC 7500/μL; platelet count 200,000/μL. Electrolytes: normal. Urinalysis: normal. ANA positive, 1:2560, nucleolar pattern; anti-Scl-70 antibody negative. Chest radiograph: bibasilar interstitial infiltrates. Abdominal radiograph and CT scan: see Figure.

Question: What is the cause of the abdominal complaints in this patient with scleroderma?

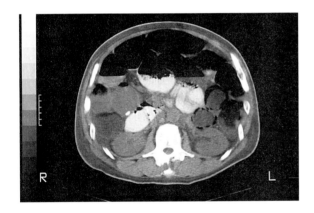

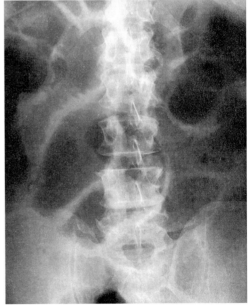

Diagnosis: Intestinal pseudo-obstruction with pneumatosis cystoides intestinalis.

Discussion: Gastrointestinal (GI) tract involvement is the most frequent visceral manifestation of systemic sclerosis (scleroderma), occurring in over 80% of patients regardless of the extent of the cutaneous disease. Multiple levels of involvement are common, with esophageal dysmotility and reflux being early, prominent features.

Small intestine complications of scleroderma include: chronic intestinal pseudo-obstruction, malabsorption, telangiectasia, and diverticuli. Scleroderma is one of the known causes of chronic intestinal pseudo-obstruction. Intestinal pseudo-obstruction leads to recurrent signs and symptoms of intestinal obstruction in the absence of mechanical obstruction of the intestinal lumen. GI manometry usually reveals decreased or absent activity fronts of the migrating motor complex. Prokinetic therapy with erythromycin and octreotide may relieve abdominal pain and nausea in some cases. Sometimes bacterial overgrowth results in intestinal distention, bloating, and malabsorption. Cyclic courses of oral antibiotics may improve diarrhea secondary to bacterial overgrowth. In severe cases of scleroderma gut disease complicated by malnutrition, total parenteral nutrition may be required.

Pneumatosis cystoides intestinalis is a rare condition defined as the presence of multiple gaseous cysts in the intestinal wall. Pneumatosis cystoides intestinalis has been associated with a variety of conditions: chronic obstructive pulmonary disease, gastric carcinoma, inflammatory bowel disease, amyloidosis, and connective tissue diseases such as lupus, juvenile arthritis, and scleroderma. In scleroderma it is seen in the setting of chronic intestinal pseudo-obstruction. Air in the bowel wall is visualized on plain radiographs with air-fluid levels (see Figure). Computed tomography may help distinguish pneumatosis intestinalis cystoides from conditions that require immediate intervention, such as abdominal abscess, bowel infarction, and mesenteric or biliary air (see Figure). Pneumatosis intestinalis cystoides may respond to conservative measures: intravenous nutritional support, antibiotics, and oxygen. In some scleroderma patients, the presence of pneumatosis cystoides intestinalis is associated with rapidly progressive disease and high mortality.

In the present case, pneumatosis cystoides intestinalis resolved with conservative management, but ultimately chronic intestinal pseudo-obstruction was complicated by severe malabsorption.

Clinical Pearls

1. The GI tract is the most frequent site of visceral involvement by systemic sclerosis (scleroderma).

2. Small intestinal complications of scleroderma include chronic intestinal pseudo-obstruction, malabsorption, telangiectasia, and diverticuli.

3. Nausea, vomiting, bloating, abdominal distention, and pain in a scleroderma patient are indicative of intestinal pseudo-obstruction.

4. Pneumatosis cystoides intestinalis occurs in scleroderma and other conditions and is defined as the presence of multiple gaseous cysts in the intestinal wall.

REFERENCES
1. Abu-Shakra, Guillemin F, Lee P. Gastrointestinal manifestations of systemic sclerosis. Semin Arthritis Rheum 1994;24:29–39.
2. Sjogren RW. Gastrointestinal motility disorders in scleroderma. Arthritis Rheum 1994;37:1265–1282.
3. Verne GN, Eaker EY, Hardy E, Sninsky CA. Effect of octreotide and erythromycin on idiopathic and scleroderma-associated intestinal pseudoobstruction. Digest Dis Sci 1995;40:1892–1901.
4. Quiroz ES, Flannery MT, Martinez EJ, Warner EA. Pneumatosis cystoides intestinalis in progressive systemic sclerosis: a case report and literature review. Am J Med Sci 1995;310:252–255.

PATIENT 58

A 68-year-old man with nocturnal low back pain

A 68-year-old man had a 6-month history of nocturnal low back pain with recumbency. The pain was dull, aching, and had a boring quality. Salicylates provided no relief. He denied fever, night sweats, weight loss, or GI or GU symptoms. Aside from the night-time pain, he felt well and could exercise without difficulty. His past history was remarkable for coronary artery disease; he had had a transurethral resection of his prostate.

Physical Examination: Temperature 97.5°; heart rate 82; respirations 18; blood pressure 172/80. General: healthy appearance and in no acute distress. HEENT: normal. Chest: clear. Cardiac: normal. Abdomen: normal. Rectal: normal. Neurologic: normal. Back: nontender. Extremities: normal.

Laboratory Findings: WBC 7500/μL; Hct 40%; platelet count 200,000/μL. ESR: 16 mm/hr. Electrolytes: normal. Calcium, phosphorus, alkaline phosphatase: normal. SPEP: normal. PSA: 0.9 IU/mL. Spine MRI and bone scan: see Figure.

Question: What is the most likely cause of the patient's nocturnal back pain?

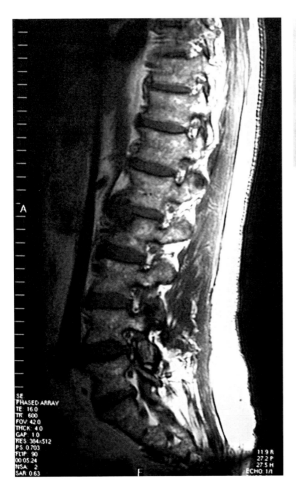
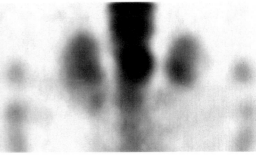

Diagnosis: Schmorl (cartilaginous) node.

Discussion: Nocturnal pain classically is associated with bone tumors, either benign or malignant. Malignant bone lesions produce pain of persistent and increasing intensity. Localized tenderness may be present, as well as neurologic signs if nerve roots or the spinal cord is compressed. Constitutional signs and symptoms often accompany bone pain from malignant neoplasms.

Benign neoplasms also may cause nocturnal pain or pain with recumbency. Usually there are no systemic signs or symptoms. Osteoid osteoma is a common benign tumor of bone that classically produces nocturnal pain. The peak incidence of osteoid osteoma is in young adults, aged 20 to 30 years, but some osteoid osteomas may present in childhood or in the elderly. Long bones of the lower extremity are involved most frequently, but bones of the hands, feet, and spine also may be affected. Approximately 7% of osteoid osteomas occur in the spine, usually in the lumbar vertebrae. The posterior elements are involved more frequently than the vertebral body. In the spine, osteoid osteomas may be associated with nonstructural scoliosis. An osteoid osteoma appears radiographically as a centrally located, round or oval radiolucent area measuring less than 1.5 cm in diameter, surrounded by a zone of uniform bone sclerosis. The lesion avidly accumulates bone-seeking radiopharmaceutical agents, so bone scans demonstrating increased uptake may confirm the diagnosis and aid preoperative localization.

Another benign condition producing back pain is intervertebral disk displacement. If the nucleus pulposus herniates inferiorly or superiorly, it forms a cartilaginous (Schmorl) node. The following conditions are associated with cartilaginous nodes: intervertebral (osteo-) chondrosis, Scheuermann disease (juvenile kyphosis), trauma, hyperparathyroidism, osteoporosis, infection, and neoplasm. MR imaging is valuable for assessing abnormalities at the discovertebral junction and shows high signal intensity on T2-weighted images (see Figure). In symptomatic cases there is inflammation and edema in the vertebral bone marrow that may produce increased uptake on bone scan (see Figure). After healing of endplate fracture and subsidence of inflammation, the Schmorl node becomes asymptomatic.

The present patient had a symptomatic Schmorl node, confirmed by MRI and bone scan findings. Osteoid osteoma was less likely in view of the patient's age, location of the lesion, and failure to respond to salicylates. Over the next 6 months the pain gradually subsided.

Clinical Pearls

1. Tumors of the spine cause pain at night or with recumbency.

2. Osteoid osteoma is a benign bone tumor that usually presents in young adults and most frequently affects long bones.

3. Relief of nocturnal pain with salicylates supports the diagnosis of osteoid osteoma.

4. Cartilaginous (Schmorl) node is disk material that herniates inferiorly or superiorly and is another benign condition that produces low back pain.

5. Conditions associated with Schmorl nodes include intervertebral (osteo-) chondrosis, Scheuermann disease (juvenile kyphosis), trauma, hyperparathyroidism, osteoporosis, infection, and neoplasm.

REFERENCES

1. Healey JH, Ghelman B. Osteoid osteoma and osteoblastoma. Current concepts and recent advances. Clin Orthop 1986;204:76–85.
2. Resnick D, Niwayama G. Degenerative disease of the spine. In: Resnick D, Niwayama G (eds): Diagnosis of Bone and Joint Disorders, vol 6. Philadelphia, WB Saunders, 1988, pp 1481–1561.
3. Borenstein DG. Low back pain. In Klippel JH, Dieppe PA (eds): Rheumatology. London, Mosby, 1994.
4. Hamanishi C, Kawabata T, Yosii T, et al. Schmorl's nodes on magnetic resonance imaging. Their incidence and clinical relevance. Spine 1994;19:450–453.
5. Kakitsubata Y, Nabeshima K, Kakitsubata S, et al. Discovertebral junction of the spine—a cadaveric study by spin-echo MR imaging. Acta Radiol 1995;36:1–8.
6. Takahashi K, Miyazaki T, Ohnari H, et al. Schmorl's nodes and low-back pain. Analysis of magnetic resonance imaging findings in symptomatic and asymptomatic individuals (abstr). Eur Spine J 1995;4:56–59.

PATIENT 59

A 38-year-old man with chronic back pain and stiffness

A 38-year-old man had a longer than 10-year history of low back pain and stiffness. Symptoms began insidiously with no history of trauma. Pain and stiffness were worse in the morning and improved with exercise. Over the years he noted progressive stiffness of the back with inability to touch his toes. There was no history of peripheral joint, cutaneous, ocular, oral, gastrointestinal, or genitourinary symptoms.

Physical Examination: Vital signs: normal. General examination: normal. Musculoskeletal: full range of motion of peripheral joints; loss of lumbar lordosis with tender paraspinal muscles; Schöber test reduced to 1 cm; chest expansion 2.5 cm; normal cervical spine mobility.

Laboratory Findings: WBC 7500/μL; Hct 40%; platelet count 225,000/μL; ESR 30 mm/hr. Chemistries: normal. Urinalysis: normal. Sacroiliac radiographs: complete bony ankylosis of each sacroiliac joint. Lumbar spine radiographs: see Figure.

Question: What radiographic findings are characteristic of this disease?

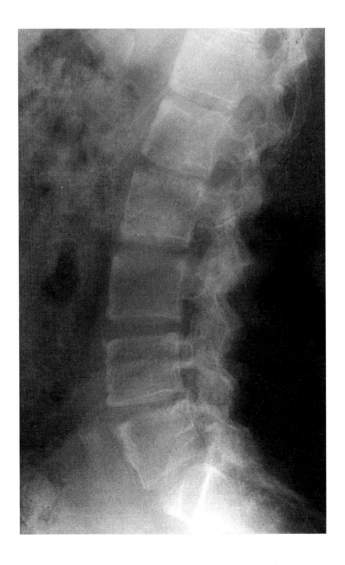

Answer: Ankylosing spondylitis with radiographic findings of "shiny corners," vertebral squaring, and syndesmophytes.

Discussion: Ankylosing spondylitis (Gr. = *anky-los,* "bent" and *spondylos,* "spine") is a chronic inflammatory disease that primarily affects the axial skeleton and is strongly associated with the presence of HLA B-27. By definition the sacroiliac joints are inflamed, and sacroiliitis is often the earliest finding in adults with ankylosing spondylitis. The normal undulating articular surface of the sacroiliac joint makes radiographic evaluation difficult, but the best method is an anteroposterior radiograph taken with the tube angulated 25 to 30 degrees cephalad. Bilateral and symmetric changes occur, including periarticular osteoporosis, erosions, subchondral sclerosis and later bony ankylosis. As the disease progresses, inflammation and bony changes occur in the spine (see below) from the lumbosacral region to the thoracic and cervical spine.

A history of persistent, dull, lower back pain insidious in onset and accompanied by morning stiffness is typically obtained from patients with ankylosing spondylitis, usually males in their second or third decade. Extraarticular symptoms, such as enthesitis (inflammation of the muscular or tendinous attachment to bone) and acute iritis are common, whereas aortic insufficiency, apical pulmonary fibrosis, and cauda equina syndrome are rare.

Physical findings often are confined to the axial skeleton and may be subtle in early cases. Pain from sacroiliitis may be elicited by direct pressure over the joints, compression of the pelvis with the patient lying on his side, or downward pressure on the flexed knee and contralateral anterior superior iliac spine with the hip flexed, abducted, and externally rotated. Loss of lordosis and limited forward flexion of the lumbar spine develop with progression of the disease. The latter is defined by an abnormal Schöber test: less than 5 cm increase in the distance between the "dimples of Venus" at level of the spinous process of L5 and a mark 10 cm superiorly in the midline with forward flexion.

Radiographic signs of spinal involvement may be seen at the discovertebral junctions, apophyseal joints, costovertebral joints, posterior ligamentous attachments, and atlantoaxial joint. Osteitis at the anterior margin of the discovertebral junction is an early feature. Reparative new bone formation results in loss of the normal concavity, creating a "squared" contour to the vertebral body (see Figure). Erosion at the discovertebral junction is known as the Romanus lesion, which heals with reactive sclerosis, producing a "shiny corner" (see Figure). Vertical osseous outgrowths that eventually extend across the intervertebral disks, "syndesmophytes," represent ossification of the anulus fibrosus (see Figure).

Management of ankylosing spondylitis involves patient education, physical therapy, and nonsteroidal anti-inflammatory drugs. In the present case, there was significant improvement in pain and stiffness with physical therapy and indomethacin.

Clinical Pearls

1. The diagnosis of ankylosing spondylitis should be considered in a young man with chronic low back pain of insidious onset and with more than 1 hour of morning stiffness.

2. Early findings of sacroiliitis on physical examination include pain when the sacroiliac joint is stressed and an abnormal Schöber test, respectively.

3. The normal undulating articular surface of the sacroiliac joint makes radiographic evaluation difficult, but the best method is an anteroposterior radiograph taken with the tube angulated 25 to 30 degrees cephalad.

4. Radiographic features of spinal involvement include "shiny corners," squaring of the vertebra, and syndesmophytes.

REFERENCES

1. Bywaters EGL. Pathology of the spondyloarthropathies. In: Calin A (ed): Spondyloarthropathies. Orlando, Grune & Stratton, 1984, pp 43–68.
2. Guerra J Jr, Resnick D. Radiographic and scintigraphic abnormalities in seronegative spondyloarthropathies and juvenile chronic arthritis. In: Calin A (ed): Spondyloarthropathies. Orlando, Grune & Stratton, 1984, pp 339–381.
3. Khan MA, Vander Linden SR. Ankylosing spondylitis and associated diseases. Rheum Dis Clin North Am 1990;16:551–579.
4. Ramos-Remuc C, Russell AS. New clinical and radiographic features of ankylosing spondylitis. Curr Opin Rheumatol 1992;4:463–469.
5. Ramos-Remuc C, Russell AS. Clinical features and management of ankylosing spondylitis. Curr Opin Rheumatol 1993;5:408–413.

PATIENT 60

A 65-year-old man with arthritis, splenomegaly, and neutropenia

A 65-year-old man with a 10-year history of erosive arthritis presented with fever and cellulitis. His rheumatoid arthritis had been treated with NSAIDs and gold salts with a good response. He denied recent joint swelling or morning stiffness. In the past, he had leg ulcers and two episodes of bronchopneumonia.

Physical Examination: Temperature 101.2°; pulse 80; respirations 14; blood pressure 120/80. Skin: subcutaneous olecranon nodules; cellulitis of the right leg. HEENT: normal. Chest: clear. Cardiac: normal. Abdomen: spleen palpable 5 cm beneath left costal margin. Neurologic: normal. Musculoskeletal: symmetric, deforming arthritis involving PIP, MCP, wrist, knee, and MTP joints. Extremities: healed malleolar ulcers and hyperpigmentation of legs.

Laboratory Findings: WBC 3800/μL with 95% lymphocytes and 5% neutrophils; peripheral smear (see Figure); Hct 32%; platelets 102,000/μL. RF 1:1280; ANA 1:80. Serum protein electrophoresis: polyclonal hyperglobulinemia. Bone marrow: maturation arrest at myelocyte stage and focal lymphoid infiltrate.

Question: What is the hematologic complication in this patient with rheumatoid arthritis?

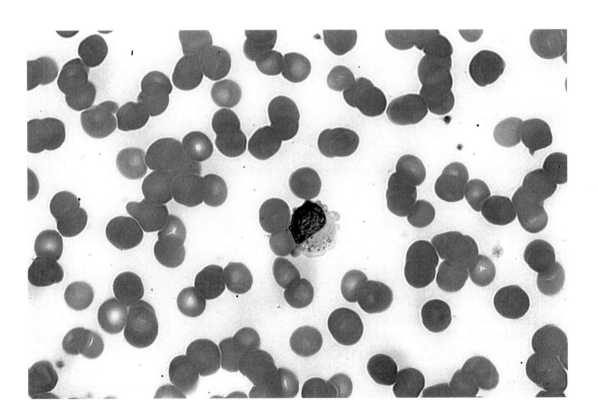

Answer: Felty syndrome with large granular lymphocyte expansion.

Discussion: Felty syndrome, a triad of rheumatoid arthritis (RA), splenomegaly, and neutropenia, occurs in approximately 1% of RA patients. Other manifestations of Felty syndrome are leg ulcers, hyperpigmentation, lymphadenopathy, and thrombocytopenia. Felty syndrome usually occurs in patients with chronic, seropositive, erosive, and nodular RA, but the synovitis may not be active when features of Felty syndrome are present. Bone marrow examination is essential to exclude drug-induced cytopenias; the characteristic finding in Felty syndrome is maturation arrest at the myelocyte stage, adequate megakaryocytes, and focal lymphoid infiltrates.

Up to one-third of Felty syndrome patients have an increased number of large granular lymphocytes (LGL) on peripheral blood smear. These LGLs contain azurophilic cytoplasmic granules (see Figure) and express T cell and NK cell surface antigen markers (usually CD3+ CD8+ CD57+), but they exhibit decreased NK activity. RA patients with LGLs have the same HLA-DR4 background seen in RA patients with or without Felty syndrome, which differs from that of LGL syndrome patients without arthritis.

Recurrent infection may complicate Felty syndrome. Splenectomy may or may not improve neutropenia and generally is not recommended. Felty syndrome may improve with disease-modifying drugs, such as gold salts or methotrexate. Lithium carbonate may improve the neutropenia by demarginating white blood cells. Granulocytopenia also may improve with granulocyte colony stimulating factor (GCSF), but arthritis flare and leukocytoclastic vasculitis have been reported following this therapy.

The present patient's cellulitis resolved with antibiotic therapy. Gold was discontinued, and neutropenia improved with low-dose weekly methotrexate. Large granular lymphocytosis persisted without evidence of transition to LGL leukemia on long-term follow-up.

Clinical Pearls

1. Felty syndrome, the triad of rheumatoid arthritis (RA), splenomegaly, and neutropenia, occurs in approximately 1% of patients with RA.

2. Felty syndrome usually occurs in the setting of chronic, seropositive, erosive RA with nodules, but synovitis may not be active when Felty syndrome presents.

3. Up to one-third of Felty syndrome patients have an increased proportion of large granular lymphocytes (LGL) on peripheral blood smear.

4. Expanded populations of large granular lymphocytes in RA patients usually express T-cell and NK-cell surface antigen markers, but exhibit reduced NK activity.

5. Recombinant human granulocyte colony stimulating factor (GCSF) may increase the neutrophil count of Felty syndrome patients, but arthritis flare and leukocytoclastic vasculitis may complicate GCSF therapy.

REFERENCES

1. Wallis WJ, Loughran TP Jr, Kadin ME, et al. Polyarthritis and neutropenia associated with circulating large granular lymphocytes. Ann Intern Med 1985;103:357–362.
2. Barton JC, Prasthofer EF, Egan ML, et al. Rheumatoid arthritis associated with expanded populations of granular lymphocytes. Ann Intern Med 1986;104:314–323.
3. Bowman SJ, Sivakumaran M, Snowden N, et al. The large granular lymphocyte syndrome with rheumatoid arthritis. Immunogenetic evidence for a broader definition of Felty's syndrome. Arthritis Rheum 1994;37:1326–1330.
4. Vidarsson B, Geirsson AJ, Onundarson PT. Reactivation of rheumatoid arthritis and development of leukocytoclastic vasculitis in a patient receiving granulocyte colony-stimulating factor for Felty's syndrome. Am J Med 1995;98:589–591.

PATIENT 61

A 65-year-old man with back pain and azotemia

A 65-year-old man presented with a 3-month history of back pain. The pain was constant and dull and did not radiate. There was no history of trauma. It was accompanied by low-grade fever and a 10-pound weight loss.

Physical Examination: Temperature 100.2°; pulse 80; respirations 16; blood pressure 140/90. Skin: normal. HEENT: arcus senilus. Chest: clear. Cardiac: S4 gallop. Abdomen: midabdominal bruit. Back: no CVA or spine tenderness. Neurologic: normal. Musculoskeletal: normal. Extremities: 1+ edema in legs.

Laboratory Findings: WBC 12,000/μL; Hct 38%; platelets 300,000/μL; ESR 110 mm/hr. BUN 70 mg/dL; Cr 3.8 mg/dL. Urinalysis: normal. RF and ANA: negative. Abdominal ultrasound: 4-cm aortic aneurysm and bilateral hydronephrosis. CT scan: retroperitoneal mass encircling and obstructing the ureters. Biopsy of the mass: see Figure.

Question: What diagnosis can explain the patient's back pain and renal failure?

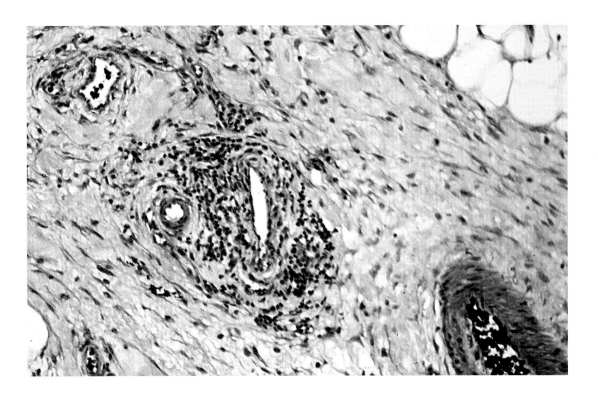

Answer: Retroperitoneal fibrosis.

Discussion: Retroperitoneal fibrosis (Ormond disease) is a rare condition predominantly affecting patients 40 to 60 years of age and often associated with atherosclerosis of the aorta. Diagnosis is often delayed because of the nonspecific nature of presenting symptoms, eg, pain in the back, flank or abdomen. Less frequent symptoms include weight loss, malaise, leg swelling, claudication, hematuria, Raynaud phenomenon, and oliguria. Physical examination is often unrevealing, but 5 to 10% of patients with retroperitoneal fibrosis will have an abdominal or rectal mass. Laboratory tests usually are consistent with inflammation and azotemia: elevated ESR or C-reactive protein, normochromic and normocytic anemia, leukocytosis, thrombocytosis, and elevated serum creatinine.

When considering the diagnosis of retroperitoneal fibrosis, abdominal CT or MRI scans should be obtained. Findings suggestive of retroperitoneal fibrosis include the presence of a retroperitoneal mass surrounding the aorta and medial deviation of the ureters with proximal ureteral obstruction and hydronephrosis. The fibrotic mass may extend or be accompanied by mediastinal fibrosis, or it may extend to the small bowel, pancreas, spinal cord, and inferior vena cava. A related condition, idiopathic fibrosclerosis, is characterized by fibrotic masses in the orbits, Reidel thyroiditis, mediastinal fibrosis, and fibrotic arthropathy.

The histopathology of retroperitoneal fibrosis typically involves a central core of bland fibrosis with an inflammatory reaction at the leading edge of the mass. The mixed inflammatory cell infiltrate is composed of macrophages, lymphocytes, plasma cells, and eosinophils (see Figure); macrophages are often lipid-laden. Vasculitis is seen in 10% of lesions (see Figure). Although the pathogenesis is poorly understood, one hypothesis considers retroperitoneal fibrosis to be a complication of chronic periaortitis. Indeed, many patients with retroperitoneal fibrosis show an abnormal antibody response to ceroid, a complex of proteins and oxidized LDL, suggesting an immune response to components of atherosclerotic plaques.

Other conditions associated with retroperitoneal fibrosis include: drugs (methysergide, beta blockers, ergot alkaloids, methyldopa, hydralazine), malignancy (sarcoma, lymphoma, or metastastic cancer of lung, breast, etc.), infections (tuberculosis, histoplasmosis), ankylosing spondylitis, PAN, Wegener granulomatosis, SLE, systemic sclerosis, and Crohn disease.

Once the diagnosis of retroperitoneal fibrosis has been confirmed, high-dose corticosteroid therapy, eg, prednisone, 1 mg/kg/d, is the primary treatment. Most patients have an excellent response to steroid therapy. Some patients require urinary drainage by stent placement, which can be removed when the mass shrinks with therapy. Other immunosuppressive drugs, such as azathioprine and cyclophosphamide, have been effective in some cases, and recent reports of response to tamoxifen are intriguing.

In the present patient, ureteral obstruction was relieved by percutaneous stent placement, and there was complete recovery following high-dose corticosteroid therapy.

Clinical Pearls

1. Retroperitoneal fibrosis, Ormond disease, is a rare cause of back pain, flank pain, or abdominal pain.

2. Consider the diagnosis of retroperitoneal fibrosis in a middle-aged or elderly patient with the triad of abdominal and/or back pain, elevated ESR, and weight loss.

3. The diagnosis of retroperitoneal fibrosis can be confirmed by CT or MRI scans.

4. Vasculitis of small and medium-sized vessels is seen in 10% of biopsy specimens of retroperitoneal fibrosis.

5. The mainstay of therapy for retroperitoneal fibrosis is high-dose corticosteroids and urinary tract drainage; some patients may respond to immunosuppressive drugs or tamoxifen.

REFERENCES

1. Loffeld RJLF, van Weel Th F. Tamoxifen for retroperitoneal fibrosis. Lancet 1993;341:382.
2. Keith DS, Larson TS. Idiopathic retroperitoneal fibrosis. J Am Soc Nephrol 1993;3:1748–1752.
3. Hughes D, Buckley PJ. Idiopathic retroperitoneal fibrosis is a macrophage-rich process. Implications for its pathogenesis and treatment. Am J Surg Pathol 1993;17:482–490.
4. Gilkeson GS, Allen NB. Retroperitoneal fibrosis. A true connective tissue disease. Rheum Dis Clin North Am 1996;22:23–38.
5. Moncure AC, Nielsen GP. A 31-year-old woman with lumbar and abdominal pain, hypertension, and a retroperitoneal mass (Case 27–1996). Case Records of the Massachusetts General Hospital. N Engl J Med 1996;335:650–655.

PATIENT 62

A 75-year-old woman with arthritis and hand weakness

A 75-year-old woman had seropositive rheumatoid arthritis for more than 20 years. Treatment with nonsteroidal antiinflammatory agents, prednisone, gold salts, and methotrexate provided only moderate control of her disease over the years. For the past 6 months she noticed weakness and numbness of her hands. She denied lower extremity weakness and urinary or bowel incontinence.

Physical Examination: Temperature 99.5°; blood pressure 132/78; pulse 88; respirations 16. Musculoskeletal system: cervical spine had diminished range of motion in rotation, extension, and lateral flexion; shoulder abduction limited to 70 degrees bilaterally; elbows had bilateral 15-degree flexion contractures; wrists were fused; hands had ulnar deviation and diffuse thenar, hypothenar, and interosseous wasting; grip strength was significantly diminished. Neurologic: biceps, triceps, and brachioradialis reflexes 1+ and symmetric; sensation to light touch and pinprick reduced in the fingers and hands.

Laboratory Findings: CBC, electrolytes, and urinalysis: normal. Cervical spine MRI: (see Figure).

Question: What is the diagnosis and potential complication?

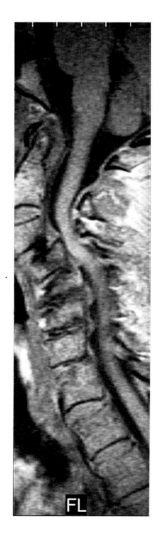

Answer: Rheumatoid arthritis with subaxial subluxation and spinal cord compression.

Discussion: Symptomatic spinal involvement in rheumatoid arthritis is uncommon, occurring in fewer than 10% of cases. Its occurrence is nearly always limited to patients with long-standing seropositive disease. Symptoms depend on the site of instability or cord compression.

The spinal lesion most characteristic of RA is atlantoaxial subluxation. Synovial proliferation causes erosion and disruption of the longitudinal ligament that approximates the odontoid process to the posterior aspect of the anterior arch of C2. Atlantoaxial subluxation may be detected by lateral cervical spine radiographs in flexion and extension. When the neck is held in extension, normally there is a minimum space (up to 3 mm) between the anterior aspect of the odontoid and the posterior aspect of the anterior arch of C1. In RA, however, this space may be exaggerated with measurements exceeding 3 mm. Significant asymptomatic increase in C1–C2 subluxation is sometimes possible because the spinal canal is relatively wide at this level and the odontoid process may be eroded. Greater subluxation (10 to 15 mm) is usually symptomatic.

Cervical subluxation should be considered in any RA patient who complains of neck or occipital pain, a jerking sensation when the neck is flexed, paresthesias of arms or legs, dizziness, or ataxia. Physical findings may include weakness in the extremities, diminished sensation (particularly vibration and proprioception) and pathological reflexes. Particular care must be taken with such patients to avoid spinal cord compression, either as a result of trauma or manipulation, as for example during intubation for general anesthesia. Radiography of the cervical spine should be obtained with flexion and extension views to screen for atlantoaxial and subaxial subluxation. MRI scanning is helpful since impingement of the spinal cord can be visualized (see Figure).

Cervical spine problems other than C1–C2 subluxation my occur in RA. Destruction of the lateral masses of C1 results in tilting of the head to one side or intrusion of the odontoid process into the foramen magnum. The latter can result in compression of the medulla with resultant syncope, dizziness, or apnea. The cervical spine may be involved at areas more caudal to C1–C2, ie, subaxial subluxation. These lesions occur most commonly at C3–C4 or C4–C5.

Treatment of cervical subluxation varies according to severity. For patients with neurologic symptoms surgical fixation should be undertaken to preclude spinal cord or medullary compression. Surgical approaches are directed toward fixation to maintain the spinal canal and reduce motion of the affected vertebrae relative to one another. Therefore, both posterior and anterior approaches have been undertaken. The best results have been obtained with fusion of C1 to the occiput to C2 in cases of axial subluxation, and of the involved vertebrae when the subluxation is subaxial. Prolonged postoperative immobilization with either halo fixation or a Strijker circoelectric frame is usually required.

The present patient was treated with anterior fusion of the involved vertebral bodies with screw fixation. A prolonged hospitalization for rehabilitation was required for her to return to functional status.

Clinical Pearls

1. Cervical subluxation in rheumatoid arthritis occurs most commonly in women with seropositive, erosive disease of long duration.

2. Cervical spine disease in rheumatoid arthritis most commonly occurs at the level of C1 and C2, where erosion of the odontoid and destruction of the ligament which opposes the odontoid to the posterior aspect of C1 results in widening of the intervening space.

3. Symptoms of cervical subluxation include neck and occipital pain, paresthesias of extremities, weakness, and bladder or bowel incontinence.

4. Magnetic resonance imaging (MRI) is the most useful technique to demonstrate impingement on the spinal cord.

5. Surgical treatment of cervical subluxation should be undertaken in symptomatic patients with cord compression and is aimed at fusion of vertebral bodies and posterior elements.

REFERENCES

1. Bland JH. Rheumatoid subluxation of the cervical spine. J Rheumatol 1990; 17:134–137.
2. Agarwal AK, Peppelman WC, Kraus DR, Eisenbeis CH. The cervical spine in rheumatoid arthritis. BMJ 1993, 306:79–80.
3. Rosa C, Alves M, Queiros MV, et al. Neurologic involvement in patients with rheumatoid arthrits with atlantoaxial subluxation. J Rheumatol 1993;20:248–252.

PATIENT 63

A 38-year-old woman with knee pain and dystrophic nails

A 38-year-old woman had a lifelong history of bilateral knee pain and dystrophic fingernails. At age 12 she dislocated first one and then the other patella, each of which was found to be hypoplastic. She went on to experience chronic knee pain, as well as elbow and shoulder pain. Dystrophic fingernails were present at birth. Her father had similar nails and chronic knee pain.

Physical Examination: Vital signs: normal. Skin: normal. Nails: bilateral dystrophy with splitting and triangle-shaped lunulae (see Figure). HEENT: normal. Chest: clear. Cardiac: normal. Abdomen: normal. Neurologic: normal. Musculoskeletal: small patellae with lateral subluxation; elbow flexion contractures; limited shoulder range of motion.

Laboratory Findings: CBC, ESR, RF, electrolytes, BUN and creatinine: normal. Knee radiographs: see Figure. Pelvis films: iliac horns.

Question: What is the genetic disorder manifested by this patient?

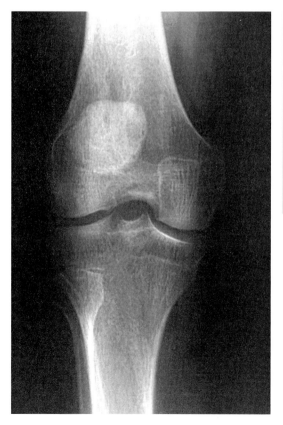

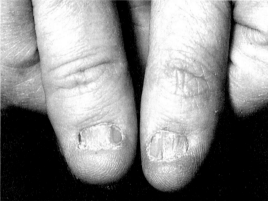

Answer: Osteo-onychodysplasia (nail-patella syndrome).

Discussion: Osteo-onychodysplasia, or nail-patella syndrome (Fong syndrome) is an autosomal dominant disorder characterized by: (1) dystrophic fingernails and toenails; (2) hypoplastic or absent patella; (3) iliac horns; and (4) radial head dysplasia. Other features variably present include renal insufficiency and sensorineural hearing loss.

Nails may be absent, but more often are hypoplastic or dysplastic. Nail changes, which are bilateral and symmetric, include discoloration, splitting, and longitudinal pterygion (see Figure). Triangular lunulae are pathognomonic of nail-patella syndrome. The patella may be absent or hypoplastic with a tendency to lateral subluxation. Clinical manifestations usually occur in the second and third decades. Radial heads may be hypoplastic and associated with Madelung deformity. Abnormalities of the knees, elbows, and other joints lead to chronic arthralgia and arthritis. A pathognomonic feature of nail-patella syndrome is the presence of iliac horns, which are symmetric bony protrusions arising from the posterior ilium or anterior superior iliac crest. Clavicular horns also have been described.

Renal disease occurs in approximately 50% of nail-patella syndrome patients to a variable degree between and within families. Proteinuria, hematuria, and hypertension are commonly observed. Light microscopy may be normal, but electron microscopy reveals irregular thickening of the glomerular basement membrane with electron lucent areas and collagen deposition. End-stage renal disease develops in approximately 30% of cases in their early 30s.

The genetic abnormality in nail-patella syndrome is located on the long arm of chromosome 9. This is also the chromosomal location of COL5A1, the gene for the alpha chain of type V collagen. Although once believed to be the gene for nail-patella syndrome, recent genetic mapping has excluded COL5A1 as the candidate gene.

There is no specific therapy for the nail-patella syndrome. Chronic joint disease may require arthroplasty. Renal failure may necessitate renal transplantation, and the glomerular lesion does not recur in the transplanted kidney.

In the present patient chronic joint disease led to arthroplasty of the knee, hip, and shoulder joints. Renal function has remained normal.

Clinical Pearls

1. Osteo-onychodysplasia, the nail-patella syndrome, is characterized by the tetrad: (1) dysplastic fingernails and toenails; (2) hypoplastic or absent patella; (3) iliac horns; and (4) hypoplastic radial heads.

2. The nail-patella syndrome is an autosomal dominant disorder, the gene defect of which maps to chromosome 9.

3. Nail changes are bilateral and symmetric and include discoloration, splitting, longitudinal pterygium and triangular lunulae.

4. A pathognomonic radiographic finding of nail-patella syndrome is an iliac horn.

5. Glomerulopathy occurs in 50% of nail-patella patients and results in renal failure in 30%.

REFERENCES

1. Resnick D. Additional congenital or heritable anomalies and syndromes. In: Resnick D, Niwayama G (eds): Diagnosis of Bone and Joint Disorders. Philadelphia, WB Saunders, 1988, pp 3541–3600.
2. Ioan DM, Maximilian C, Fryns JP. Madelung deformity as a pathognomonic feature of the onycho-osteodysplasia syndrome. Genet Couns 1992;3:25–29.
3. Greenspan DS, Northrup H, Au KS, et al. COL5A1: fine genetic mapping and exclusion as candidate gene in families with nail-patella syndrome, tuberous sclerorsis 1, hereditary hemorrhagic telangieactasia, and Ehlers-Danlos syndrome type II. Genomics 1995;25:737–739.
4. Yarali HN, Erden GA, Karaarslan F, et al. Clavicular horn: another bony projection in nail-patella syndrome. Pediatr Radiol 1995;25:549–550.

PATIENT 64

A 56-year-old man with hemolysis and renal failure

A 56-year-old man was well until 6 months previously, when he developed reversible, cold-induced color changes in his hands. He was found to have pitting scars on his fingertips and color changes consistent with Raynaud phenomenon. After testing revealed anemia and a positive antinuclear antibody test, prednisone 60 mg per day was initiated. He became progressively weaker and was transferred for care.

Physical Examination: Temperature 98.4°, pulse 94, respirations 22, blood pressure 144/92. Skin: pitting scars on several fingertips that were also tapered. Chest: bibasilar rales. Heart: S4 gallop. Abdomen: normal. Extremities: trace edema. Microscopic nailfold capillary examination: avascular areas and dilated loops.

Laboratory Findings: WBC 9400/μL, HCT 29%, platelets 66,000/μL. Peripheral smear: see Figure. Na^+ 138 mEq/L; K^+ 4.6 mEq/L; HCO_3^- 18 mEq/L; Cl^- 98 mEq/L; BUN 98 mg/dL; Cr 6.3 mg/dL. Urinalysis: 100 mg/dL protein, 3^+ hemoglobin, 4–5 RBC/hpf, 2–3 WBC/hpf. Chest radiograph: slightly enlarged cardiac silhouette, increased interstitial markings and blunting of the right costophrenic angle. A kidney biopsy was performed: see Figure.

Question: What is the diagnosis?

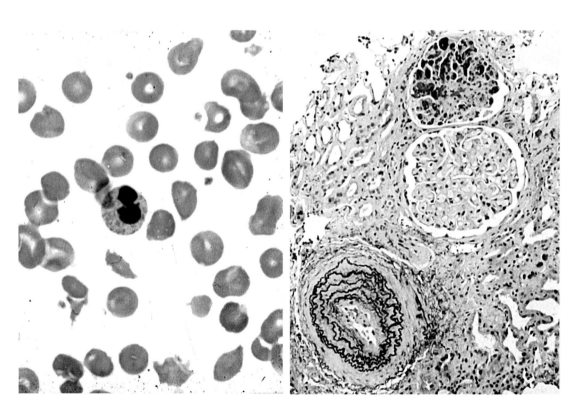

Answer: Normotensive scleroderma renal failure.

Discussion: Renal involvement in patients with scleroderma generally occurs early in the course of the illness (mean of 3.2 years after onset). Most patients have the diffuse cutaneous variant of the disease and are in a phase of progressive dermal thickening. The onset of renal disease may be explosive, with extreme hypertension, headache, blindness, oliguria, and edema, a syndrome termed "scleroderma renal crisis." As in the current patient, however, the onset of renal failure is not necessarily accompanied by hypertension and is termed "normotensive renal failure."

Renal failure results from vascular abnormalities affecting the renal arterioles. Luminal narrowing results from intimal proliferation and diminishes blood flow, with resultant renin release from the juxtaglomerular apparatus. Renin produces further vasoconstriction via angiotensin II. Thus, a cycle is perpetuated that results in cortical ischemia and necrosis. Examination of the blood smear may demonstrate fragmented erythrocytes and thrombocytopenia that result from shear forces in the renal vessels.

Until recently the development of renal disease in scleroderma meant rapid and irreversible loss of renal function accompanied by uncontrollable hypertension. New developments, particularly the discovery of angiotensin converting enzyme (ACE) inhibitors, have changed the prospects of such patients. While these medications have made the onset of renal disease less ominous, the recognition of early signs of hypertensive renal crisis is even more critical now, because early treatment can prevent the worst complications. Any elevation in blood pressure should be taken seriously in a scleroderma patient. Even pressure rises from low-normal levels that remain in the normotensive range ($< 140/90$ mmHg) should prompt evaluation for renal disease.

During the early stages of treatment, captopril is recommended because of its short half-life and flexibility of dosage. For those who remain hypertensive, captopril should be maintained and other antihypertensive agents added. Calcium-channel blockers and α-adrenergic blockers are most commonly used. Antihypertensive therapy should be maintained even if renal failure ensues, because some patients may improve their renal function sufficiently to discontinue dialysis. Despite the major advance in therapy that ACE inhibitors have afforded, a substantial number of patients still progress to renal failure. Dialysis can be accomplished either by hemodialysis or by peritoneal dialysis. Renal transplantation has been successful in patients with scleroderma without recurrence of disease in the transplanted kidney.

The onset of renal failure without hypertension (normotensive) has been noted in a small subset of scleroderma patients. This syndrome is associated with myositis, glucocorticoid treatment, microangiopathic hemolysis and thrombocytopenia. The prognosis is poorer than for those with hypertensive crisis. It is not known whether ACE inhibitors are effective, but the authors' experience with two patients would suggest they may not provide any benefit.

In the present patient, end-stage renal failure occurred despite therapy with ACE inhibitors. He was maintained on hemodialysis until death ensued from a myocardial infarction.

Clinical Pearls

1. Scleroderma renal disease usually is characterized by acute hypertension and renal failure ("scleroderma renal crisis") early in the course of the disease in patients with diffuse cutaneous systemic sclerosis.

2. Scleroderma renal crisis is best managed with ACE inhibitors that block the production of angiotensin, which results from high renin production.

3. Normotensive scleroderma renal failure is associated with myositis, glucocorticoid therapy, microangiopathic hemolysis, and thrombocytopenia. Treatment with ACE inhibitors appears less effective than in hypertensive scleroderma renal crisis, but is still recommended.

REFERENCES
1. Helfrich DJ, Banner B, Steen VD, et al. Normotensive renal failure in systemic sclerosis. Arthritis Rheum 1989;32:1128–1134.
2. Steen VD, Costantino JP, Shapiro AP, et al. Outcome of renal crisis in systemic sclerosis: relation to availability of angiotensin converting enzyme (ACE inhibitors). Ann Intern Med 1990;113:352–357.
3. Donohoe JF. Scleroderma and the kidney. Kidney Int 1992;41:462–477.

PATIENT 65

A 3-year-old girl with arthritis and red eye

A 3-year-old girl had painful swelling of the left index finger and left great toe that began at 17 months of age. Initial eye examination was normal, but at age 2½ years her mother reported a 1-week history of a red eye. There was no history of trauma, fever, rash, or diarrhea. The father had an unknown type of arthritis, and a paternal uncle had ankylosing spondylitis.

Physical Examination: Vital signs: normal. Skin: normal. HEENT: 1+ circumcorneal injection OD with hazy anterior chamber and posterior synechiae on slit lamp exam; semi-opaque band extending across cornea (see Figure). Chest: clear. Cardiac: normal. Abdomen: normal. Neurologic: normal. Musculoskeletal: fusiform swelling of left index finger PIP joint and sausage-like swelling of left first and second toes.

Laboratory Findings: WBC 7900/μL; Hct 37.5%; platelet count 343,000/μL. ESR: 20 mm/hr. ANA: positive, 1:80, homogeneous pattern. RF: negative. HLA B-27: positive.

Question: What are the ocular complications of this child's disease?

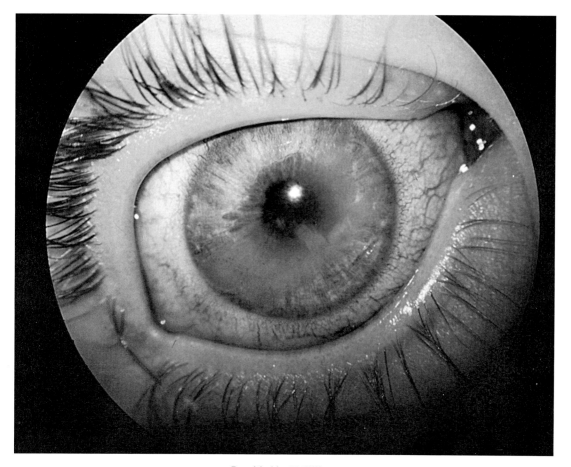

Provided by E. Wilson

Diagnosis: Pauciarticular juvenile chronic arthritis with anterior uveitis, band keratopathy, and posterior synechiae.

Discussion: Juvenile chronic arthritis (also known as juvenile rheumatoid arthritis or juvenile arthritis) is the most common connective tissue disease of childhood. The etiology and pathogenesis are poorly understood. Six consecutive weeks of objective synovitis in one or more joints is required for diagnosis, plus exclusion of other conditions that may present with chronic arthritis. Examples of diseases that may mimic juvenile arthritis include: systemic lupus erythematosus and other connective tissue diseases; chronic infections such as Lyme disease or tuberculosis; malignancies such as neuroblastoma or leukemia; and various immunodeficiency states. There are no diagnostic tests for juvenile chronic arthritis. Correct diagnosis is dependent on a complete history and physical examination plus exclusion of other conditions.

Three distinct types of disease onset are recognized. Children are classified based on the first 6 months of disease as: (1) systemic-onset (Still disease); (2) polyarticular onset ($\geq$ 5 joints involved); or (3) pauciarticular onset ($\leq$ 4 joints involved). Monoarticular arthritis is considered part of the pauciarticular subset, but infection is a strong consideration in any patient with monoarthritis. Systemic-onset JRA accounts for 10% of cases, occurs at any age, and is characterized by high fever, evanescent salmon-pink rash, leukocytosis, hepatosplenomegaly, and lymphadenopathy. Polyarticular onset JRA accounts for about 40% of cases, affects girls more than boys (2:1), and is seropositive (RF+) in only a minority of cases, usually adolescent girls. Pauciarticular onset JRA is the most common subset of juvenile chronic arthritis, accounting for approximately 50% of cases. This subset is further divided into two types: (1) early childhood onset, female preponderance, frequently positive ANA and negative RF; and (2) older age onset, male preponderance, ANA and RF negative, and HLA B-27 often present. Many of the latter cases represent juvenile onset spondyloarthropathy.

Ocular inflammation develops in children with JRA, almost always in those with pauciarticular onset. Chronic anterior uveitis is most likely to occur in girls with early childhood onset, pauciarticular JRA who are ANA positive. In most cases (90%) uveitis is diagnosed after development of arthritis. Uveitis is often asymptomatic at onset, detected only by slit lamp examination. Uveitis may become symptomatic later in the course of disease with decreased visual acuity. Redness and pain are rare in such children, occurring more commonly in later onset and the subset characterized by HLA B-27.

Slit lamp examination is imperative in children with JRA, especially in those with pauciarticular disease with ANA. Cells and protein haze within the anterior chamber and a punctate keratitic precipitate are the ophthalmologic signs of uveitis. Chronic inflammation leads to posterior synechiae, glaucoma, and cataract. Band keratopathy, a semiopaque band across the cornea, is a degenerative change that occurs less frequently now that uveitis is recognized and treated early, and is virtually pathognomonic of JRA. Less common ocular complications of JRA are keratoconjunctivitis sicca and corneal melt.

Successful treatment of chronic uveitis hinges on early detection by slit lamp examination. ANA-positive, pauciarticular onset children should be screened every 3 to 4 months for a period of 7 years, after which intervals between screening may be extended. Uveitis is treated with topical steroids and mydriatic agents. Band keratopathy is treated with topical chelation therapy.

The present patient had early age onset, pauciarticular arthritis with a weakly positive ANA. A number of findings actually suggest juvenile onset spondyloarthropathy: acute uveitis; sausage toes; positive family history, and positive HLA B-27. Arthritis responded to NSAIDs and low-dose, weekly methotrexate. Band keratopathy was treated with topical chelation and uveitis with steroid and atropine drops.

Clinical Pearls

1. Juvenile chronic arthritis (JCA) is defined as synovitis in one or more joints of at least 6 weeks' duration, with exclusion of other conditions that may present with arthritis.

2. Pauciarticular onset ($\leq$ 4 joints affected) is the most common type of JCA, accounting for 50% of all cases.

3. Two types of pauciarticular JCA are recognized: (1) early age onset, usually female, often ANA-positive; and (2) later age onset, usually male, HLA B-27 often present.

4. Chronic arterior uveitis, which is usually asymptomatic at onset, occurs predominantly in girls with JCA who are ANA-positive and have pauciarticular onset.

5. Complications of chronic arterior uveitis include posterior synechiae, glaucoma, cataract, and band kerotopathy.

6. All JCA patients require screening slit lamp examination, the frequency of which depends on the type of disease onset (pauci > poly > systemic) and ANA status (positive > negative).

REFERENCES

1. Rosenberg AM, Oen KG. The relationship between ocular and articular disease activity in children with juvenile rheumatoid arthritis and associated uveitis. Arthritis Rheum 1986;29:797–800.
2. Kanski JJ. Uveitis juvenile chronic arthritis: Incidence, clinical features and prognosis. Eye 1988;2:641–645.
3. Cassidy JT, Levinson JE, Brewer EJ Jr. The development of classification criteria for children with juvenile rheumatoid arthritis. Bull Rheum Dis 1989;38:1–6.
4. Kanski JJ. Uveitis in juvenile chronic arthritis. Clin Exp Rheumatol 1990;8:499–503.

PATIENT 66

A 32-year-old woman with a bullous skin rash

A 32-year-old woman was well until 2 months previously, when she developed a symmetric poly-arthritis of the small and large joints. Over-the-counter anti-inflammatory drugs provided some relief. One month later she developed bullous skin lesions, first on the trunk then spreading to involve the extremities and buccal mucosa.

Physical Examination: Temperature 99.5°; pulse 88; respiratory rate 16; blood pressure 145/84. Skin: diffuse bullae ranging from 0.5 to 3 cm in diameter with positive Nikolsy sign (splitting of skin with lateral pressure). HEENT: bullae on buccal mucosa. Chest: clear. Cardiac: normal. Extremities: swelling and tenderness of wrists, metacarpophalangeal, proximal interphalangeal, knee, ankle, and metatarsopha-langeal joints.

Laboratory Findings: WBC 12,500/μL with 63% PMNs, 32% lymphocytes, 5% monocytes; Hct 32%; platelets 231,000/μL. Na^+ 142 mEq/L; K^+ 4.4 mEq/L; Cl^- 98 mEq/L, HCO_3^- 23 mEq/L. BUN 19 mg/dL, Cr 1.1 mg/dL. Urinalysis: normal. Chest radiograph: normal. ECG: normal. Antinuclear antibody: positive, 1:1280 with a homogeneous pattern; anti-double stranded DNA antibodies: positive, 1:1280. C3: 63 mg/dL (83–178); C4: undetectable. Anticardiolipin antibodies: IgG 19 (0–15), IgM 23 (0–15). Lupus anticoagulant: positive. Antibodies to type VII collagen: positive. Skin biopsy: see Figure.

Question: What is the diagnosis?

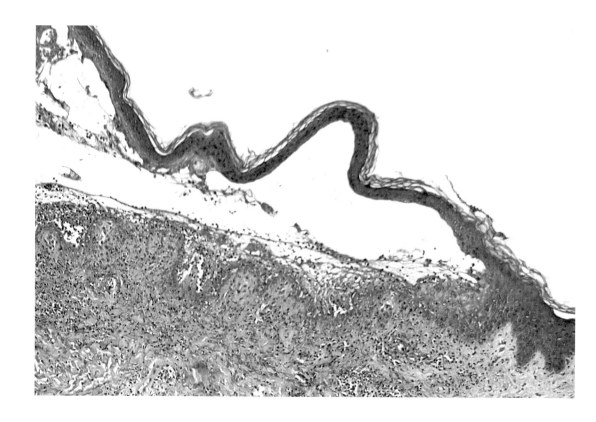

Diagnosis: Bullous lupus erythematosus.

Discussion: Cutaneous eruptions occur in the majority of patients with systemic lupus erythematosus (SLE) (55 to 85% in large series) and is the presenting complaint in 30 to 40%. Of the various eruptions seen in SLE, the most common is a malar rash (the familiar butterfly pattern), which occurs in 30 to 60% of patients. The classic butterfly rash is an erythematous and papulosquamous eruption over the cheeks and nasal bridge. The occurrence of the butterfly rash correlates with systemic disease activity. Other conditions that cause butterfly pattern eruptions on the face include acne rosacea and seborrheic dermatitis.

Discoid lesions are the second most common type of skin eruption in SLE, occurring in 15 to 30% of patients and as the presenting complaint in about 10%. These lesions begin as flat macules or papules with a scaly surface and evolve into erythematous plaques covered with an adherent scale. Plaques may enlarge and coalesce to form large, disfiguring lesions. Discoid lesions occur most commonly on the face, scalp, ears, and extensor surfaces of the arms.

Bullous skin lesions are much less common in SLE, occurring in only 1 to 2% of patients, usually with evidence of active systemic disease. Bullous lupus must be distinguished from primary vesiculobullous disease, eg, bullous pemphigoid, herpes zoster, dermatitis herpetiformis, and epidermolysis bullosa acquisita. Bullous LE ranges from only a few blisters to a severe, generalized eruption with extensive areas of denuded skin resembling toxic epidermal necrolysis. The histology of bullous LE is a neutrophilic infiltration with microabscess formation in the dermal papillae. Direct immunofluorescence shows deposits of IgG and complement components in the basement membrane area. The antigenic target in these lesions is type VII collagen, a major component of the basement membrane. The same antigen is recognized in epidermolysis bullosa acquisita. Circulating antibodies to type VII collagen can be demonstrated in most patients with bullous LE lesions using sensitive ELISA techniques.

Treatment of bullous LE may be difficult. Systemic corticosteroids often are ineffective. The addition of immunosuppressive drugs (azathioprine, cyclophosphamide, cyclosporin) may be beneficial, but there are no large series to prove their efficacy. Dapsone, useful against other types of neutrophilic inflammation, has been reported to ameliorate bullous LE. Dapsone must not be given to patients with deficiency of glucose-6-phosphate dehydrogenase because of the likely development of hemolysis in such patients. Dapsone is initiated at 50 mg per day and increased to 100 mg per day once tolerance of the drug is evident. Blood counts must be monitored closely in patients taking dapsone. Although plasmapheresis has been used to treat bullous LE, such treatment has not been shown to be effective despite evidence of circulating anti-collagen VII antibodies.

The present patient had SLE with the characteristic arthritis, bullous skin lesions, positive tests for ANA, anti-double stranded DNA, and anti-type VII collagen. Low levels of serum C3 and C4 reflected ongoing complement consumption. Treatment with high doses of systemic corticosteroids, dapsone, and oral cyclophosphamide improved her skin lesions, but a cerebrovascular accident, probably a result of the lupus anticoagulant, resulted in death.

Clinical Pearls

1. The most common skin lesions in SLE are a malar rash and discoid lesions, but other skin eruptions can occur, including diffuse bullous disease.

2. Bullous LE most commonly occurs in patients with evidence of active systemic disease, anti-double stranded DNA antibodies, and low serum complement levels.

3. Patients with bullous LE often have circulating anti-type VII antibodies, the antigenic target in bullous LE.

4. Because neutrophils play a prominent role in the inflammation of bullous LE, dapsone may be useful.

5. When using dapsone care must be taken to ascertain the patient's level of glucose-6-phosphate dehydrogenase, because dapsone may precipitate a hemolytic reaction in those deficient in G6PD.

REFERENCES
1. Camisa C. Vesiculobullous systemic lupus erythematosus. A report of four cases. J Am Acad Dermatol 1988;18:93–100.
2. Olansky AJ, Briggaman RA, Gammon WR, et al. Bullous systemic lupus erythematosus. J Am Acad Dermatol 1982;4:511–520.
3. Lindsov R, Reymann F. Dapsone in the treatment of cutaneous lupus erythematosus. Dermatologica 1986;4:214–217.
4. Fleming HG, Bergfeld WF, Tomecki KJ, et al. Bullous systemic lupus erythematosus. Int J Dermatol 1989;28:321–326.

PATIENT 67

A 55-year-old woman with chest pain and hypotension

A 55-year-old woman noticed anterior chest pain for the previous 2-week period and reported a 2-month history of low grade fever and fatigue. Over the past week she had exertional dyspnea and worsening chest discomfort. There was no radiation of the pain, but there was a change in intensity when she changed position. On the day of presentation she was unable to stand because of dizziness. Her only medication was thyroid hormone replacement.

Physical Examination: Temperature 100.5°; pulse 110; blood pressure 78/42, with a paradoxic pulse of 18 mmHg. Skin: faint erythematous rash over the cheeks. Chest: dullness to percussion at the left base; bibasilar rales. Cardiac: distended jugular veins, soft S1 and S2, two-component friction rub over the precordium. Abdomen: liver span 14 cm. Extremities: 1+ pretibial edema.

Laboratory Findings: WBC 12,500/μL with 82% neutrophils, 16% lymphocytes, 2% monocytes; Hct 29%; platelets 211,000/μL. Electrolytes normal; BUN 23 mg/dL, Creatinine 0.9 mg/dL. Urinalysis: trace protein, 0–2 RBCs/hpf. ANA: positive, 1:1280, peripheral pattern. ECG: ST segment elevation. Chest radiograph: see Figure.

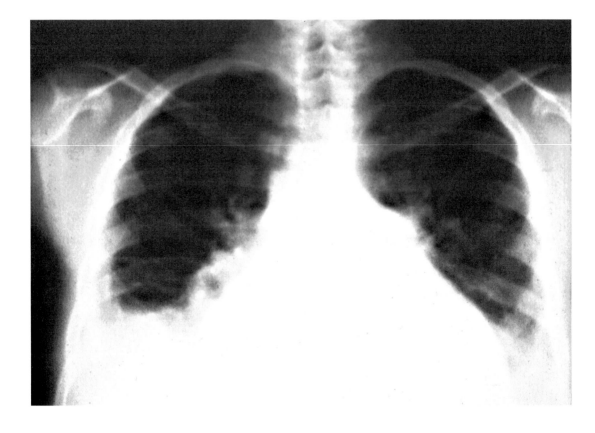

Question: What is the cause and treatment for this patient's hypotension?

Diagnosis: Systemic lupus erythematosus with pericardial effusion and tamponade.

Discussion: The most common cardiac abnormality in SLE is pericardial involvement. Although autopsy studies show pericardial involvement in 80% of SLE cases, clinically evident pericarditis is found in only about 20 to 40% of patients in large series. Pericardial fluid found by echocardiography is often asymptomatic. When symptomatic, the classic feature of pericardial disease in SLE is the same as from any other cause: anterior chest pain that varies with position. In SLE there is frequently an accompanying pleural effusion (see Figure). Physical examination may disclose a pericardial friction rub.

Pericardial effusion is an infrequent presenting manifestation of SLE. When it is noted, the diagnosis of SLE rests on the presence of other symptoms or signs of the disease as well as a positive test for serum antinuclear antibodies.

Pericardial fluid in SLE is typically exudative, with a nucleated cell count of 3000 to 5000/μL. Although ANA and LE cells frequently are present in the pericardial fluid, testing the fluid lends no additional benefit to serum testing. Indeed, when the diagnosis of SLE is known or confirmed by serologic testing, pericardiocentesis for diagnostic purposes is unnecessary.

Treatment of SLE pericarditis with NSAIDs usually is sufficient to control symptoms and resolve the effusion. Corticosteroid treatment may be necessary for resistant disease or when large effusions are present. The occurrence of tamponade is infrequent in SLE, and aspiration of fluid for therapeutic purposes should be undertaken if tamponade has occurred. Surgical creation of a pericardial "window" sometimes is necessary to treat recurrent pericardial effusion. Treatment with immunosupressive drugs (azathioprine or cyclophosphamide) and also with high-dose intravenous immunogolbulin have been reported to be helpful in controlling disease resistant to conservative management.

The present patient underwent emergency aspiration of 300 mL pericardial fluid for relief of tamponade. Treatment with prednisone (60 mg/day) was initiated, and the pericardial effusion resolved in two weeks. Later, hydroxychloroquine was added when she developed a discoid rash and arthralgia.

Clinical Pearls

1. Symptomatic pericarditis occurs in 20 to 40% of SLE patients but rarely progresses to tamponade.

2. Symptomatic pericardial effusion in SLE often is accompanied by pleural effusion.

3. Diagnostic pericardiocentesis is rarely required except when other features of SLE are lacking, but aspiration may be required to treat tamponade.

4. Treatment of lupus pericarditis with nonsteroidal anti-inflammatory drugs usually is sufficient to relieve pain and reduce pericardial effusion. Corticosteroids sometimes are required, and a pericardial "window" may be necessary to treat recurrent effusions.

REFERENCES

1. Kelly TA. Cardiac tamponade in systemic lupus erythematosus. An unusual manifestation. South Med J 1987;80:514–515.
2. Hjortkjoer Peterson H, Nielsen H, Hansen M, et al. High dose immunoglobulin therapy in pericarditis caused by SLE. Scand J Rheumatol 1990;19:91–93.
3. Crozier IG, Li E, Milne MJ, Nicholls M. Cardiac involvement in systemic lupus erythematosus detected by echocardiography. Am J Cardiol 1990;65:1145–1148.

PATIENT 68

A 3-year-old girl with arthritis and a photosensitive rash

A 3-year-old girl presented with a 6-month history of fever up to 106°F, an evanescent erythematous rash, and joint pain with morning stiffness. On initial evaluation, she was noted to be febrile and irritable with splenomegaly and an erythematous, maculopapular rash on the trunk. Initial laboratory investigations revealed leukocytosis, anemia, elevated ESR (107 mm/hr), and negative RF and ANA. Evaluation for infection was negative, and a diagnosis of systemic-onset juvenile rheumatoid arthritis (Still's disease) was made. Treatment with naproxen (15 mg/kg/d) resulted in marked improvement, and she did well until the following summer when she presented with a blistering skin rash and scarring in light-exposed areas. She was taking no other medications. Her grandmother had systemic lupus erythematosus.

Physical Examination: Temperature 98.3°F, pulse 116, respirations 18, blood pressure 88/60. Skin: fair-skinned child with multiple scars on dorsum of the hands and forearms; superficial scars and blisters on the face (see Figure). Nodes: negative. HEENT: normal. Chest: clear. Cardiac: normal. Abdomen: normal. Neurologic: normal. Musculoskeletal: full range of motion without synovitis.

Laboratory Findings: WBC 6,000/μL; Hct 40.2%; platelets 263,000/μL; ESR 4 mm/hr. Chemistries: normal. RF and ANA: negative. Quantitative stool coproporphyrin, urinary uroporphyrin and erythrocyte protoporphyrin: normal.

Question: What is the cutaneous complication in this child with JRA?

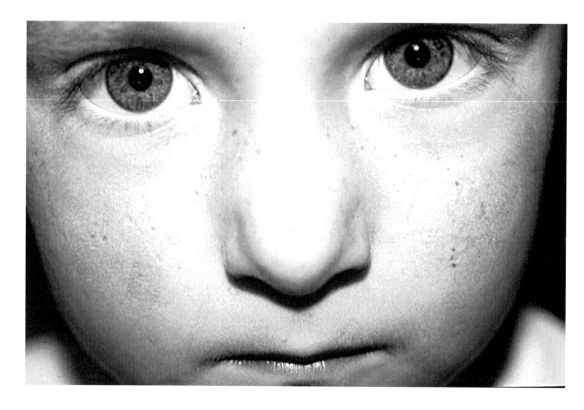

Diagnosis: Naproxen-induced pseudoporphyria.

Discussion: Rash is one of the classic extra-articular manifestations of systemic-onset juvenile rheumatoid arthritis, or Still's disease. The rash is an erythematous, macular (2–5 mm) eruption that occurs most commonly on the trunk and proximal extremities but may occur on the face, palms, or soles. The rash is evanescent and nearly always present during febrile episodes, which typically occur once daily (quotidian) or twice daily (double quotidian). Individual lesions resolve in a few minutes or hours without scarring. Skin lesions may be precipitated by rubbing or scratching the skin, the Köbner phenomenon.

Pseudoporphyria is a cutaneous disorder characterized by skin fragility, vesiculation, and scarring in light-exposed areas occuring in the presence of normal porphyrin metabolism. Histology of this photo-induced blistering disorder resembles that of porphyria cutanea tarda. Pseudoporphyria can be induced by a number of drugs, including nonsteroidal antiinflammatory drugs (NSAIDs).

Naproxen is a phenylpropionic acid NSAID frequently used to treat JRA in children. Approximately 10% of JRA patients in some series develop pseudoporphyria while taking naproxen. Erythema, vesiculation, or increased skin fragility complicated by scarring of sun-exposed skin may also be seen (see Figure). Pseudoporphyria, shallow facial scars, and skin fragility occur much less frequently with other NSAIDs. Children with fair skin and blue eyes are particularly at risk. All findings except scarring resolve within 6 months after discontinuation of naproxen.

Other causes of photodermatitis, such as porphyria or SLE, must be excluded. In the present case there was no biochemical or serologic abnormality to suggest other causes. Ibuprofen was prescribed, and the skin fragility and blisters resolved within two weeks of discontinuing naproxen.

Clinical Pearls

1. The rash of systemic-onset JRA (Still's disease) is an erythematous, macular eruption that occurs most commonly on the trunk and proximal extremities.

2. The rash is often present during the high (quotidian) fever, can sometimes be precipitated by rubbing or scratching the skin (the Köbner phenomenon), and fades without scarring.

3. In any child with a blistering rash, skin fragility, or shallow facial scars, one should consider disorders of porphyrin metabolism, such as porphyria cutanea tarda.

4. Pseudoporphyria is a complication of the NSAID naproxen, occurring in more than 10% of JRA patients treated with this drug.

5. The lesions of naproxen-induced pseudoporphyria resolve with cessation of the drug.

REFERENCES

1. Silver RM. Nonsteroidal anti-inflammatory drugs in the management of juvenile arthritis. J Clin Pharmacol 1988;28:566–570.
2. Wallace CA, Farrow D, Sherry DD. Increased risk of facial scars in children taking nonsteroidal antiinflammatory drugs. J Pediatr 1994;125:819–822.
3. Lang BA, Finlayson LA. Naproxen-induced pseudoporphyria in patients with juvenile rheumatoid arthritis. J Pediatr 1994; 124:639–642.
4. Creemers MC, Chang A, Franssen MJ, et al. Pseudoporphyria due to naproxen. A cluster of 3 cases. Scand J Rheumatol 1995;24:185–197.
5. Girschick HJ, Hamm H, Ganser G, et al. Naproxen-induced pseudoporphyria: Appearance of new skin lesions after discontinuation of treatment. Scand J Rheumatol 1995;24:108–111.

PATIENT 69

A 67-year-old man with leg numbness and eosinophilia

A 67-year-old man noticed numbness that began in his toes and progressed to the feet, distal legs, and fingertips over a 3-month period. He experienced postprandial, mid-abdominal pain during this period and lost 20 pounds. Recently, he noticed several raised, erythematous lesions over both shins. There was a history of asthma for 15 years treated with inhaled sympathomimetic drugs and occasional courses of oral corticosteroids.

Physical Examination: Temperature 97.4°F, pulse 76, blood pressure 100/60, respirations 18, weight 134 pounds. Skin: several 2 to 6 mm raised, purpuric pretibial lesions. HEENT: temporal wasting. Chest: scattered expiratory wheezes. Heart: normal. Abdomen: right upper quadrant tenderness, no organomegaly. Musculoskeletal: no synovitis. Neurological: diminished perception of light touch in feet, distal legs, and fingers.

Laboratory Findings: WBC 18,400/μl with 33% neutrophils, 58% eosinophils, 9% lymphocytes; HcT 36%; ESR 139 mm/hour. Electrolytes: normal. Bilirubin 0.8 mg/dL; AST 164 IU/L (17–59); LDH 1412 IU/L (313–618); albumin 3.2 g/dL. Hepatitis B and C serologies: negative. Cryoglobulin: 9 mg/dL, containing IgG, IgM, IgA, C1q. SPEP: polyclonal hypergammaglobulinemia. Biopsy of skin lesion: see Figure.

Questions: What is the diagnosis and how should the patient be treated?

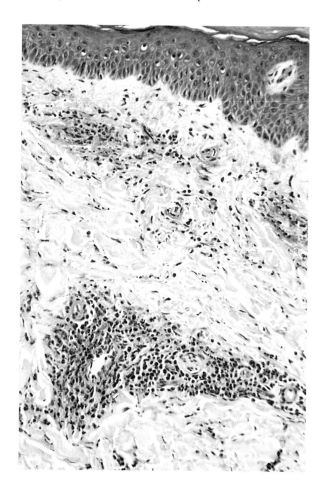

Diagnosis: Churg-Strauss vasculitis.

Discussion: Vasculitis of small and medium-sized vessels causes manifestations in multiple organs. Constitutional symptoms include fatigue, weight loss, and fever. The most commonly occurring skin lesion is palpable purpura caused by leukocytoclastic vasculitis. In these lesions, small blood vessels are infiltrated by polymorphonuclear leukocytes with prominent destruction of the blood vessel wall. These lesions can be associated with a number of conditions, including polyarteritis nodosa, Henoch-Schönlein purpura, mixed cryoglobulinemia, drug hypersensitivity, hypocomplementemic vasculitis, and connective tissue diseases, particularly Sjögren syndrome.

Types of vasculitis are distinguished by historical features, size of the involved blood vessels, and laboratory tests. The occurrence of vasculitis in a patient with a history of asthma and blood eosinophilia is characteristic of Churg-Strauss vasculitis, also known as allergic angiitis and granulomatosis. This condition, which is more common in men than women, occurs only in adults with an average age of onset of 45 to 50 years. When the vasculitis occurs, asthma has usually been present for 5 to 10 years.

The initial symptoms of Churg-Strauss vasculitis usually are weight loss and fever. Two-thirds of patients have cutaneous lesions, including subcutaneous nodules, palpable purpura, and digital infarctions. Abdominal symptoms are uncommon but occasionally result from granulomatous vasculitis of the visceral vessels. Involvement of the vaso nervorum may result in a sensory peripheral neuropathy or mononeuritis multiplex. Lung involvement is radiographically evident in about 50% of cases, and there may be patchy infiltrates (Löffler syndrome), large nodular infiltrates, or diffuse interstitial lung disease. Less common manifestations include myocardial infarction due to coronary vasculitis and retinal ischemia from ophthalmic arteritis.

The characteristic laboratory finding is eosinophilia with absolute counts between 5,000 and 20,000/µl. The ESR is always elevated, and there is often an accompanying anemia. A diagnosis of Churg-Strauss vasculitis is based on clinical features supported by pathologic findings: systemic illness in a middle-aged man with a history of asthma is suggestive, as is the presence of marked eosinophilia, leukocytoclastic vasculitis of the skin, and peripheral neuropathy. The diagnosis is confirmed by histologic findings in the skin, nerve, or lung. In cases in which the clinical diagnosis is secure, lung biopsy is unnecessary. Other causes of eosinophilia which must be considered include parasitic infestation, neoplastic disease (particularly lymphoma), atopic dermatitis, and the hypereosinophilic syndrome.

Treatment of Churg-Strauss vasculitis is with high dose corticosteroids. Prednisone (1 mg/kg/day) is usually sufficient to control the symptoms. There is almost always a rapid drop in the absolute eosinophil count with such treatment. As opposed to polyarteritis nodosa or Wegener granulomatosis, treatment with cytotoxic agents usually is not required.

Biopsy of the present patient's skin lesion revealed leukocytoclastic vasculitis and a predominantly eosinophilic inflammatory infiltrate in the dermis (see Figure). Treatment was started with 60 mg/day of prednisone. Two weeks later his appetite had returned, the sedimentation rate was 18 mm/hour and the peripheral WBC was 14,600 with <1% eosinophils. Eight months later the prednisone dose was 10 mg/day, the ESR 20 mm/hour and the eosinophil count 1.6% of 7,100 nucleated cells/µL.

Clinical Pearls

1. The differential diagnosis of constitutional symptoms (fever, weight loss, malaise) in a middle-aged man with a history of asthma includes Churg-Strauss vasculitis, neoplasia, hypereosinophilic syndrome, and chronic infection.

2. The absolute peripheral eosinophil count in Churg-Strauss vasculitis is often between 5,000 and 20,000/µl.

3. The clinical manifestations of Churg-Strauss vasculitis include palpable purpura due to leukocytoclastic vasculitis, peripheral neuropathy, abdominal visceral ischemia, and pulmonary infiltrates. Less commonly, coronary arteritis may lead to myocardial infarction and ophthalmic artery involvement to blindness.

4. Eosinophilia and symptoms of Churg-Strauss vasculitis resolve rapidly with high dose corticosteroid therapy. Most cases do not require the addition of cytotoxins, but these can be used for their corticosteroid-sparing effect.

REFERENCES

1. Chumbley LC, Harrison EG, DeRemee RA. Allergic granulomatosis and angiitis (Churg-Strauss syndrome): Report and analysis of 30 cases. Mayo Clin Proc 1977;52;477–489.
2. Kattah JC, Chrousos GA, Katz PA, et al. Anterior ischemic optic neuropathy in Churg-Strauss syndrome. Neurology 1994;44:2200–2202.
3. Kozak M, Gill EA, Green LS. The Churg-Strauss syndrome. A case report with angiographically documented coronary involvement and a review of the literature. Chest 1995;107:578–580.
4. Sehgal M, Swanson JW, DeRemee RA, Colby TV. Neurologic manifestations of Churg-Strauss syndrome. Mayo Clin Proc 1995;70:337–341.
5. Chen KR, Su WP, Pittelkow MR, Leiferman KM. Eosinophilic vasculitis syndrome: Recurrent cutaneous eosinophilic necrotizing vasculitis. Semin Dermatol 1995; 14:106–110.

PATIENT 70

A 45-year-old man with arthritis and nail pits

A 45-year-old man presented with a 6-month history of arthritis affecting one knee and one wrist. Joint pain and swelling was preceded by the recurrence of pits in the fingernails. He denied skin rash, eye symptoms, or back pain. There was no family history of arthritis or skin disease.

Physical Examination: Vital signs: normal. Skin: 1 cm diameter plaque of scaly skin in the gluteal fold; nails: see Figure. Musculoskeletal: asymmetric oligoarthritis involving the right wrist and left knee.

Laboratory Findings: WBC 8,000/μL; Hct 40%; platelets 250,000/μL; ESR 35 mm/hr. RF and ANA: negative. Synovial fluid: 12,000 WBC/μL with 70% neutrophils, 10% lymph, 20% monocytes. Polarizing microscopy: no crystals.

Question: What disease accounts for the arthritis and nail changes?

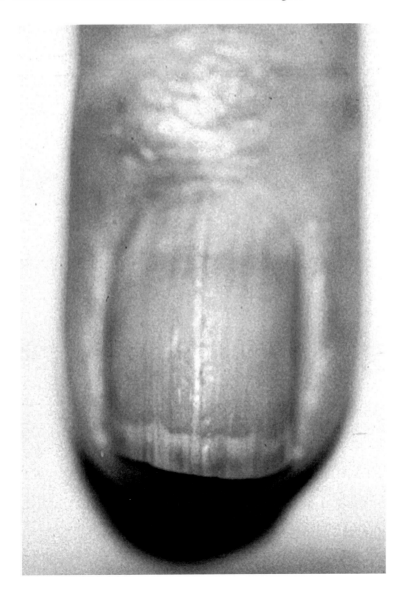

Diagnosis: Psoriasis.

Discussion: Of people with psoriasis, 6–20% develop inflammatory arthritis. Psoriatic arthritis can exist with or without skin lesions, or there may be nail involvement only. Usually psoriasis precedes the arthritis, but in some patients (15–20%) the arthritis antedates the skin lesions. Some patients with arthritis will have only mild psoriasis lying in one of the "hidden" areas such as the scalp, umbilicus, perineum, or gluteal fold.

Five subtypes of psoriatic arthritis have been recognized: (1) an asymmetrical oligoarthritis which occurs in 50% of patients with psoriatic arthritis; (2) a symmetrical polyarthritis resembling rheumatoid arthritis except for the absence of rheumatoid factor; (3) distal interphalangeal (DIP) arthritis considered classic but accounting for only 5% of cases; (4) arthritis mutilans characterized by osteolysis and dissolution of the joint leading to the "pencil-in-cup" radiographic appearance and the "opera-glass hand"; (5) spondylitis involving the cervical, thoracic, and lumbar spine often accompanied by an asymmetrical sacroiliitis and presence of HLA B-27.

Nail psoriasis is much more common than skin psoriasis alone in patients with psoriatic arthritis, occurring in over 80% of cases. Nail changes are classically associated with DIP joint arthritis but may occur in any pattern of psoriatic arthritis. Pitting of the nail is the most characteristic nail change (see Figure). More than 20 nail pits in a patient is suggestive of psoriasis as a cause for the nail dystrophy and more than 60 nail pits is unlikely to be found in the absence of psoriasis. Other nail changes in psoriasis include onycholysis, transverse ridges (Beau's lines), stippling, loss of transparency, yellowing, and subungual keratosis. Paronychial swelling, redness, and scale may be prominent (see Figure). The combination of pitting with one or more additional changes is highly suggestive of psoriasis.

In most cases of psoriatic arthritis there is no distinctive pattern of skin involvement. Psoriatic arthritis and Reiter's syndrome overlap in several manifestations. Pustular psoriasis involving the palms and soles is indistinguishable from keratoderma blennorrhagicum. The severe exfoliative or pustular form of psoriasis with rapidly progressive polyarthritis should alert the clinician to the possibility of infection with HIV.

Treatment of psoriatic arthritis can be frustrating. In some cases the skin disease flares with NSAIDs. Many rheumatologists prefer to use the NSAID meclofenamate because the skin and joints may improve with this agent. Methotrexate is indicated for erosive disease, if there is no evidence of HIV infection or alcohol abuse. Close monitoring of CBC and liver tests is necessary, and percutaneous liver biopsy may be required if liver function tests are abnormal. The present patient was treated with topical corticosteroid cream and meclofenamate, and the skin lesions and arthritis improved.

Clinical Pearls

1. There are 5 subtypes of psoriatic arthritis: asymmetric oligoarthritis, symmetrical polyarthritis, predominant DIP arthritis, arthritis mutilans, and spondylitis.

2. In 15–20% of patients, arthritis precedes the skin lesions of psoriasis.

3. Psoriasis can be found in "hidden areas" such as the scalp, umbilicus, perineum, or gluteal fold.

4. Pitting of the nail is the most characteristic nail change of psoriasis and may occur in the absence of skin lesions; other nail findings include onycholysis, transverse ridges, stippling, loss of transparency, yellowing, and subungual keratosis.

5. The possibility of HIV infection should be considered in any patient with severe exfoliative or pustular psoriasis and rapidly progressive arthritis.

REFERENCES

1. Eastmond CJ and Wright V. The nail dystrophy of psoriatic arthritis. Ann Rheum Dis 38:226–228, 1979.
2. Winchester R: Aids and the rheumatic diseases. Bull Rheum Dis 39:1–10, 1990.
3. Smiley JD: Psoriatic arthritis. Bull Rheum Dis 44:1–2, 1995.
4. Franks Jr AG: Psoriatic arthritis. In: Sontheimer RD, Provost TT, eds. Cutaneous Manifestations of Rheumatic Diseases. Baltimore, Williams and Wilkins, 1996, pp 233–241.

PATIENT 71

A 21-year-old woman with nocturnal leg pain

A 21-year-old woman had a 5 month history of unilateral knee pain. There was no history of trauma, swelling, or constitutional symptoms. The pain was described as deep, unrelated to activity, worse at night, and relieved with aspirin.

Physical Examination: Temperature 98.4°F, pulse 76, respirations 14, blood pressure 114/64. General: healthy appearance. HEENT: normal. Chest: clear. Heart: normal. Musculoskeletal: normal, without tenderness, effusion, or limited motion of the left knee.

Laboratory Findings: Hct 42%; WBC 5,600/μl; platelets 165,000/μl; ESR 18mm/hr. Electrolytes: normal. Calcium, phosphorus, alkaline phosphatase: normal. Knee radiograph: see Figure.

Question: What is the most likely cause of the patient's nocturnal knee pain?

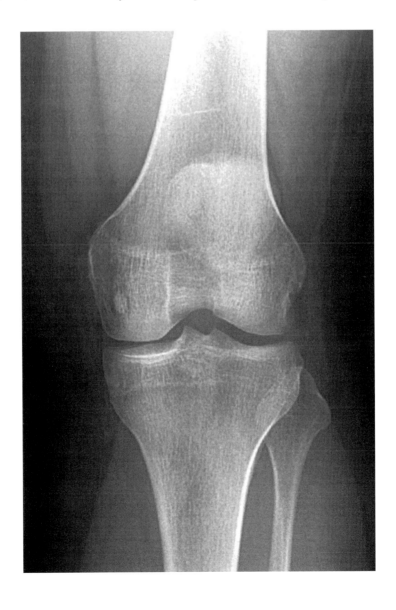

Diagnosis: Osteoid osteoma.

Discussion: In the absence of a history of trauma or systemic illness, localized bone pain must first be considered the result of neoplasia. Bone tumors, both malignant and benign, are characteristically associated with nocturnal and recumbency-induced pain. The clinical situation, location, and age of the patient are important considerations in differentiating the types of bone tumors.

The differential diagnosis of isolated bony lesions with increased radiographic opacity includes osteoma, bone island, and osteoid osteoma. Osteomas are masses of dense bone which protrude from the outer surface of bone, typically the skull, nasal sinuses, or mandible. These benign tumors are composed of dense, compact, osseous tissue. Bone islands, or enostoses, are usually asymptomatic and incidental findings on radiographs, occurring most commonly in the pelvis, ribs, and femur. In tubular bones they are most commonly located in the epiphysis or metaphysis. Such lesions are usually solitary, round or ovoid, intraosseous, sclerotic areas with discrete margins. Histologically, bone islands are composed of compact lamellar bone.

Osteoid osteomas occur primarily in children and young adults and are more common in males. The pain caused by these lesions is dull, constant, worsens at night (for unknown reasons), and is re-lieved by salicylates. When occurring in immature skeletons, osteoid osteomas may cause significant deformity. They appear radiographically as small (1.5 cm or less) round areas of sclerosis; there is often a central radiolucent area. The femur and tibia are involved most commonly, accounting for about 60% of all cases. In the spine, the lesion is usually in the posterior vertebral elements.

Bone scintigraphy is useful for distinguishing an osteoid osteoma from a bone island. While bone islands are typically "cold," osteoid osteomas universally accumulate bone-specific radiopharmaceuticals and may demonstrate a characteristic "double-density" sign: intense central activity and less intense peripheral activity. This is explained by the typical pathologic findings in osteoid osteomas: a circumscribed area of active bone formation in a highly vascular stroma surrounded by an area of more mature bone. Osteoid osteomas are benign lesions with no reported instance of malignant transformation.

Treatment of osteoid osteoma requires surgical resection of the entire central nidus. With incomplete resection, pain persists. The present patient had relief of pain with aspirin and underwent surgical resection of the osteoid osteoma after bone scintigraphy showed increased uptake. All symptoms resolved.

Clinical Pearls

1. Osteoid osteomas occur as solitary bony lesions, most commonly in the long bones of the lower extremity of children and young adults.

2. The pain of osteoid osteomas is typically dull, worsens at night, and characteristically is relieved by salicylates.

3. In contrast to radiographically similar bone islands (enostosis), osteoid osteomas accumulate bone-avid radiopharmaceuticals, often with a "double density" sign of active central uptake surrounded by a less active peripheral uptake zone.

4. Surgical resection of osteoid osteoma is curative, but any residual nidus will cause continued pain.

REFERENCES

1. Peyser AB, Makley JT, Callewart CC, et al. Osteoma of the long bones and the spine. A study of eleven patients and a review of the literature. J Bone Joint Surg Am 1996; 78:1172–1180.
2. Frassica FJ, Waltrip RL, Sponseller PD, et al. Clinicopathologic features and treatment of osteoid osteoma and osteoblastoma in children and adolescents. Orthop Clin North Am 1996;27:559–574.
3. McGrath BE, Bush CH, Nelson TE, Scarborough MT. Evaluation of suspected osteoid osteoma. Clin Orthop 1996;327:247–252.

PATIENT 72

A 15-year-old girl with knee and foot swelling

A 15-year-old girl presented with a 2-week history of painful swelling of the left foot and right knee. Pain began in the right knee, shortly after an injury during a softball game. The pain improved with NSAID therapy, but 1 week later fever of 102°F and painful swelling of the left hindfoot developed. She denied sore throat, rash, dysuria, or photophobia. She was not sexually active. She lived on a farm and was in contact with goats and cows. The patient reported an episode or diarrhea lasting 3 or 4 days, one week prior to onset of the present illness, that resolved with loperamide hydrochloride.

Physical Examination: Temperature 100.8°F, pulse 72, respirations 18, blood pressure 112/60. General appearance: well nourished teenager in no acute distress. Skin: normal. Nodes: no adenopathy. HEENT: mild conjunctival injection, OU; superficial mucosal erosion over hard palate. Chest: clear. Heart: normal. Abdomen: normal. Neurologic: normal. Musculoskeletal: synovitis of left ankle and right knee; knee flexion limited to 100°.

Laboratory Findings: WBC 9,100/μL; Hct 38.6%; platelets 248,000/μL; ESR 80 mm/hr. RF and ANA: negative. Urinalysis: normal. ASO titer: 100 IU. Synovial fluid analysis: 25 ml yellow, cloudy fluid: WBC 8,500/μL with 27% neutrophils, 43% lymphs, 30% monocytes; negative Gram stain and culture. Foot and knee radiographs: normal. Enteric pathogen serologic studies: see Table.

Serologic Studies

Organism	Titer	Reference Range
Yersinia enterocolitica	< 1:8	< 1:8
Shigella dysenteriae	< 1:8	< 1:8
Shigella flexneri	< 1:8	< 1:8
Shigella sonnei	< 1:8	< 1:8
Salmonella Ab IgG	12.9	< 5 units
Salmonella Ab IgM	29.0	< 10 units
Salmonella Ab IgA	18.5	< 10 units

Question: What is the diagnosis?

Answer: Post-dysenteric reactive arthritis.

Discussion: Reactive arthritis refers to a sterile, inflammatory synovitis occurring after an antecedent infection, usually of the genitourinary (GU) or gastrointestinal tract (GI). Organisms that have been associated with reactive arthritis include *Chlamydia,* which is a sexually-transmitted cause of urethritis or cervicitis, and *Yersinia, Salmonella, Shigella,* and *Campylobacter* species, which cause acute dysentery. Infection caused by these bacterial organisms may be followed by reactive arthritis, particularly in the immunogenetically susceptible host. Approximately 75% of patients with reactive arthritis carry the MHC class I allele, HLA-B27, compared to 7% of the normal Caucasian population of North America. Studies of point-source outbreaks of *Salmonella* enterocolitis show that up to 15% of affected individuals develop reactive arthritis. Reactive arthritis patients who are negative for HLA-B27 may carry cross-reacting group antigens.

Reactive arthritis is characterized by an asymmetric oligoarthritis, predominantly affecting the lower extremities and often accompanied by extra-articular features such as conjunctivitis and urethritis (classic Reiter's syndrome). Conjunctivitis may or may not be symptomatic. Urethritis is usually symptomatic in males, but in females cervicitis is often asymptomatic. Other features include superficial mucosal erosions of the mouth or glans penis (circinate balanitis), and keratoderma blenorrhagica.

Diagnosis of reactive arthritis demands a careful history to elicit antecedent infections of the GI or GU tracts, careful attention to the pattern of joint disease, a search for extra-articular manifestations, and exclusion of infection. Serum antibodies against enteric organisms are an adjunct to microbiologic studies and may identify the cause of reactive arthritis in cases where GI or GU symptoms have resolved. Disseminated gonococcal infection, which is the most common cause of acute arthritis in sexually active teenagers and adults, can present as oligoarthritis, tenosynovitis, dermatitis, urethritis, and conjunctivitis, and must be excluded by appropriate microbiologic studies.

Post-dysenteric reactive arthritis may resolve spontaneously within 4 months of onset, but a significant percentage of cases have chronic joint complaints and in some cases (about 15%) chronic arthritis is severe enough to require a change in work. Early antibiotic therapy does not appear to prevent the occurrence of reactive arthritis, nor does it affect its duration.

Although the present patient's GI symptoms had resolved when she presented, stool culture grew *Salmonella* species. Antibiotic therapy eradicated the *Salmonella,* but oligoarthritis persisted.

Clinical Pearls

1. Post-dysenteric reactive arthritis may follow infection by *Yersinia, Salmonella, Shigella,* or *Campylobacter* species, with the patient being free of diarrhea when arthritis presents.

2. Reactive arthritis is strongly associated with the presence of the MHC class I antigen, HLA-B27, or cross-reacting group antigens.

3. Extra-articular manifestations of reactive arthritis include conjunctivitis, uveitis, urethritis, cervicitis, dermatitis, and mucosal erosions.

4. Serum antibodies against enteric pathogens may be a useful adjunct to microbiologic cultures for establishing the cause of reactive arthritis.

5. Antibiotic therapy has not been shown to prevent reactive arthritis or to shorten the duration of the arthritis.

REFERENCES

1. Kingsley GH. Reactive arthritis: A paradigm for inflammatory arthritis. Clin Exp Rheumatol 1993;11(suppl. 8):S29–36.
2. Thomson GT, Alfa M, Orr K, et al. Serologic testing for reactive arthritis. Clin Invest Med 1994;17:212–217.
3. Locht H, Kihlstrom E, Lindstrom FD. Reactive arthritis after Salmonella among medical doctors—study of an outbreak. J Rheumatol 1994;21:371–372.
4. Thomson GT, DeRubeis DA, Hodge MA, et al. Post-Salmonella reactive arthritis: Late clinical sequelae in a point-source cohort. Am J Med 1995;98:13–21.

PATIENT 73

A 64-year-old woman with xerostomia and xerophthalmia

A 64-year-old woman gave a 15-year history of dry mouth and dry eyes. She lost her teeth due to severe dental caries. For 7 years she had intermittent, painless parotid gland enlargement, and later she was found to have painless lymphadenopathy.

Physical Examination: Temperature 98.6°F, pulse 84, respirations 16, blood pressure 134/80. Skin: no rash or nodules. Nodes: mildly enlarged, nontender cervical and supraclavicular lymph nodes. HEENT: dry conjunctiva with mucus in medial canthus; dry oral mucosa with atrophic glossitis; enlarged and nontender parotid glands (see Figure). Chest: clear. Heart: normal. Abdomen: normal. Neurologic: normal. Musculoskeletal: normal.

Laboratory Findings: WBC 3,300/µL; Hct 40.3%; platelets 300,000/µL. Serum chemistries: normal. Urinalysis normal; RF positive, 1:320; ANA positive, 1:160, homogeneous pattern; anti-SS-A and SS-B positive. Anti-ds-DNA: negative. Shirmer test: zero mm bilaterally.

Questions: What is the diagnosis and what associated malignancy should be considered?

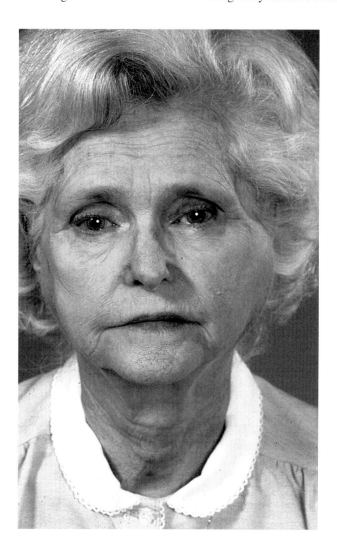

Answer: Sjögren's syndrome and non-Hodgkin's lymphoma.

Discussion: Sjögren's syndrome (SS) consists of the triad of dry mouth (xerostomia), dry eyes (xerophthalmia), and parotid gland enlargement. It is the second most prevalent autoimmune connective tissue disorder (CTD), occurring as a primary autoimmune exocrinopathy (primary SS) or as a secondary manifestation of RA, lupus, or other CTD (secondary SS).

Sjögren's syndrome occurs most commonly in middle-aged females who present with symptoms related to decreased lacrimal or salivary gland function, a condition called sicca. Xerostomia presents as oral mucosal dryness with difficulty chewing and swallowing, and painful sensation of the tongue and mouth. Loss of normal salivary flow can lead to accelerated dental caries. Xerophthalmia manifests as a dry, gritty sensation in the eyes, as well as burning, photophobia, itching, and accumulation of thick mucus in the inner canthus of the eye. Keratoconjunctivitis sicca is assessed by measurement of flow (Shirmer test) or by studies of conjunctival epithelium integrity (rose bengal staining). Less than 5 mm wetting of Shirmer test filter paper at 5 minutes is considered positive.

In Sjögren's syndrome, parotid gland enlargement is usually bilateral, painless, and intermittent. Unilateral parotid gland enlargement requires exclusion of salivary gland neoplasm. Other causes of bilateral parotid gland enlargement include viral infections (including HIV), sarcoidosis, diabetes mellitus, hyperlipidemia, hepatic cirrhosis, amyloidosis, and various drugs. Such conditions generally lack the autoimmune abnormalities seen in Sjögren's syndrome, such as RF, ANA, and anti-SS-A and SS-B antibodies. When the diagnosis is in doubt, salivary gland biopsy should be performed. Minor salivary glands in the labial mucosa can be biopsied safely. The characteristic histopathology of Sjögren's syndrome consists of focal lymphocytic infiltration and destruction of the acinar tissue.

Treatment of Sjögren's syndrome is aimed at improving mucosal dryness and preventing complications such as dental caries and corneal scarrring. Artificial saliva and tears provide symptomatic relief. Salivary flow may improve with pilocarpine. Hydroxychloroquine may be effective for some patients, improving the ESR and hypergammaglobulinemia.

Approximately 15% of Sjögren's syndrome patients have lymphadenopathy, which in some areas is quite striking (pseudolymphoma). Non-Hodgkin's B-cell lymphomas arise in some cases and may involve the salivary glands, lungs, bone marrow, and gastrointestinal tract. A fall in titer of a previously elevated rheumatoid factor (RF) may herald the transition from pseudolymphoma to lymphoma.

In the present patient, primary Sjögren's syndrome was diagnosed based on xerostomia, xerophthalmia with positive Shirmer test, parotid gland enlargement, and the absence of another CTD. Biopsy of a supraclavicular lymph node revealed histiocytosis without malignancy. Sicca improved with symptomatic therapy, and she died 6 years later from an unrelated aortic aneurysm.

Clinical Pearls

1. Sjögren's syndrome consists of dry eyes (xerophthalmia), dry mouth (xerostomia), and parotid gland enlargement. It results from an autoimmune exocrinopathy.

2. Sjögren's syndrome may occur independently (primary SS), or secondary to another CTD, such as RA or lupus (secondary SS).

3. Shirmer test < 5 mm is considered positive, but rose bengal staining with slit lamp examination is a more specific test.

4. Other conditions that may present with parotid gland enlargement include viral infections (including HIV), sarcoidosis, amyloidosis, salivary gland neoplasms, diabetes, hyperlipidemia, hepatic cirrhosis, and drug toxicity.

5. Lymphoma, usually of the non-Hodgkin's B-cell type, is a well-described complication of Sjögren's syndrome that may or may not be preceded by pseudolymphoma. Lymphoma may be heralded by a fall in RF titer.

REFERENCES

1. Foster HE, Gilroy JJ, Kelly CA, et al. The treatment of sicca features in Sjögren's syndrome: A clinical review. Br J Rheumatol 1994;33:1190.
2. Fox RI, Saito I. Criteria for diagnosis of Sjögren's syndrome. Rheum Dis Clin North Am 1994;20:391–407.
3. Fox RI. Sjogren's syndrome. Curr Opin Rheumatol 1995;7:409–416.
4. Anaya JM, McGuff HS, Banks PM, et al. Clinicopathological factors relating malignant lymphoma with Sjögren's syndrome. Semin Arthritis Rheum 1996;25:337–346.
5. Tzioufas TG. B-cell lymphoproliferation in primary Sjögren's syndrome. Clin Exp Rheumatol 1996;14(suppl):S65–70.

PATIENT 74

A 64-year-old man with rheumatoid arthritis and digital cyanosis

A 64-year-old man had a 20-year history of rheumatoid arthritis, which had been treated with injectable gold salts, NSAIDs, and prednisone. About 4 months previously he noticed small, dark areas near his fingernails, later followed by blueness of his fingertips.

Physical Examination: Temperature 99.6°F, pulse 92, respirations 16, blood pressure 132/78. Skin: cyanosis of fingertips and purple lesions on arms (see Figure). HEENT: normal. Chest: clear. Cardiac: normal. Abdomen: normal bowel sounds, no hepatosplenomegaly. Musculoskeletal: nodules over olecranon processes and in extensor tendons of several fingers; ulnar deviation at MCP joints; swelling of both wrists, knees, and ankles. Neurologic: diminished sensation of touch in a stocking and glove distribution of hands and feet.

Laboratory Findings: WBC: 8,400/µl; Hct 32%; platelets 457,000/µl; ESR 112 mm/hr. Electrolytes: normal. BUN 22 mg/dL; creatinine 1.2 mg/dL. Prothrombin time: 11 seconds. RF: positive, 1:2560. C3: 78 mg/dL (93–184), C4 9 mg/dL (15–43).

Question: What is the diagnosis?

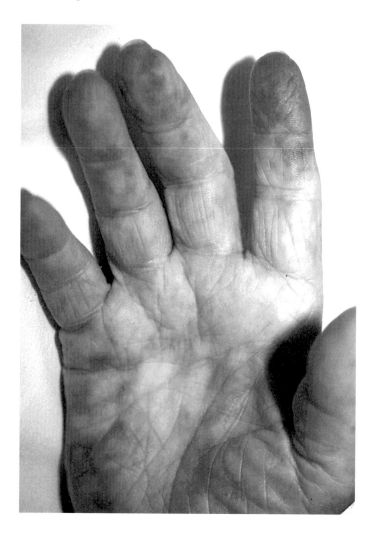

Diagnosis: Rheumatoid vasculitis.

Discussion: A variety of extra-articular manifestations are seen in rheumatoid arthritis. These include rheumatoid nodules, scleritis, Felty's syndrome, pleural or pericardial inflammation, and sicca syndrome. Vasculitis occurs in only a small fraction of RA patients, probably less than 5%, but can be severe when it occurs.

The occurrence of vasculitis in RA patients is associated with more severe, deforming arthritis, and such patients usually have a high level of rheumatoid factor. Circulating immune complexes, cryoglobulinemia, and low serum complement levels indicate that this complication of RA is mediated by deposition of immune complexes.

The clinical manifestations of vasculitis in RA patients depend on the size of the involved blood vessels. When only small vessels are involved, the manifestations are usually limited to the skin. Cutaneous involvement may take the form of palpable purpura (usually a leukocytoclastic vasculitis), ulceration of the distal legs, livedo reticularis, or periungual nailfold infarctions. Purpuric papules of the distal digital pulp (termed Bywaters' lesions) are considered to be a manifestation of mild rheumatoid vasculitis.

Arteritis of larger blood vessels is clinically indistinguishable from polyarteritis nodosa and is histologically similar as well, with inflammatory cell infiltration of all layers of the blood vessel wall, fibrinoid necrosis, and thrombosis. These vascular changes result in claudication or infarction of involved organs. Involvement of the gastrointestinal tract presents with abdominal pain after ingestion of food (abdominal angina) and may progress to infarction with perforation and/or hemorrhage. Vasculitis of the vasa nervorum results in peripheral neuropathy with sensory abnormalities or mononeuritis multiplex, such as wrist or foot drop.

Diagnosis of rheumatoid vasculitis depends upon the clinical manifestations. Laboratory tests are of limited value. The ESR is invariably elevated and early complement component levels are depressed. Biopsy of a skin lesion may show leukocytoclastic vasculitis. Peripheral nerve biopsy (e.g., the sural nerve) may demonstrate necrotizing vasculitis. Angiography of the abdominal vessels may indicate narrowing of blood vessels or pseudoaneurysm formation.

Treatment of vasculitis in RA depends upon the severity of the clinical manifestations. When limited to periungual infarctions, no treatment is indicated other than customary treatment of RA. Life-threatening ischemia of organs, however, must be treated aggressively with high-dose corticosteroids and cyclophosphamide.

The present patient had gastrointestinal involvement in addition to the digital vasculitis pictured on the preceding page. Despite corticosteroid and cyclophosphamide therapy, he died from duodenal perforation and hemorrhage.

Clinical Pearls

1. Rheumatoid vasculitis occurs in only a small subset of RA patients (probably less than 5%) who commonly have high titer rheumatoid factor.

2. Small vessel involvement may be limited to palpable purpura, periungual infarction, or digital pulp papules (Bywaters' lesions).

3. Large vessel involvement is clinically similar to polyarteritis nodosa with peripheral nerve involvement (peripheral neuropathy or mononeuritis multiplex) or visceral arteritis.

4. The diagnosis of rheumatoid vasculitis may be made on clinical grounds when manifestations are limited. Biopsy of palpable purpura usually shows leukocytoclastic vasculitis. Nerve biopsy may show vasculitis of the vaso nervosum. Abdominal angiography may show tapering of blood vessels or pseudoaneurysm formation.

5. Treatment of rheumatoid vasculitis must be appropriate for the degree of involvement. Disease limited to the digits does not require specific therapy, but large vessel involvement should be treated with high-dose corticosteroids and cyclophosphamide.

REFERENCES
1. Craig SD, Jorizzo JL, White WL, et al. Cutaneous signs of rheumatologic disease: Bywaters' lesions. Arthritis Rheum 1994;37:957–959.
2. Watts RA, Carruthers DM, Scott DG. Isolated nail fold vasculitis in rheumatoid arthritis. Ann Rheum Dis 1995;54:927–929.
3. Puechal X, Said G, Hilliquin P, et al. Peripheral neuropathy with necrotizing vasculitis in rheumatoid arthritis. A clinicopathologic and prognostic study of thirty-two patients. Arthritis Rheum 1995;38:1618–1629.
4. Voskuyl AE, Zwinderman AH, Westedt ML, et al. Factors associated with the development of vasculitis in rheumatoid arthritis: Results of a case-control study. Ann Rheum Dis 1996;55:190–192.

PATIENT 75

A 69-year-old man with a purpuric rash

A 69-year-old man developed an eruption on his forearms and legs. Oral ampicillin had been pre-scribed for pharyngitis 2 weeks prior to presentation. He was taking no other medications. The eruption was nonpruritic and occurred over a 3-day period, starting on the lower extremities and progressing to involve the thighs. He denied fever, weight loss, myalgia, paresthesias, arthralgia, abdominal pain, and hematuria.

Physical Examination: Temperature 98.8°F, pulse 82, respirations 16, blood pressure 132/78. Skin: (see Figure below left). HEENT: normal. Neck: no palpable nodes. Chest: clear. Cardiac: normal. Abdomen: normal bowel sounds, no bruits or organomegaly; stool guaiac negative. Extremities: no arthritis or edema. Neurologic: normal sensation, strength and reflexes.

Laboratory Findings: WBC 7,200/μL; Hct 38.6%; platelets 257,000/μL; ESR 53 mm/hour. PT 11.8 seconds, PTT 29 seconds. Electrolytes: normal. BUN 23 mg/dL; creatinine 1.3 mg/dL. C3: 87.9 mg/dL, C4: 22 mg/dL. AST: 23 IU/ml, total bilirubin: 1.1 mg/dL. Urinalysis: protein negative, 0–2 RBC/hpf. ANA: negative. ANCA: negative. RF: negative. Hepatitis A, B, and C serologic tests: negative. Skin biopsy: (see Figure below right); negative for IgA by immunohistochemistry.

Question: What is the diagnosis?

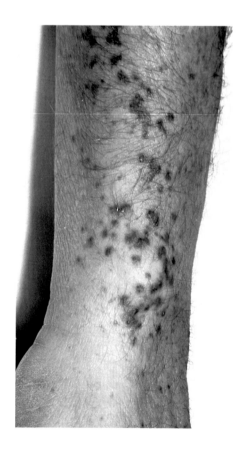

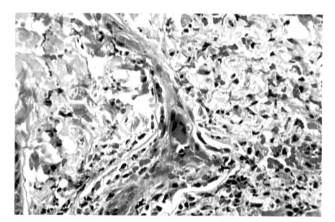

Answer: Drug-induced leukocytoclastic vasculitis.

Discussion: Vasculitis of the small vessels of the skin gives a typical clinical appearance of palpable purpura. This syndrome may occur alone or as a manifestation of a number of conditions including Henoch-Schönlein purpura, mixed cryoglobulinemia, Sjögren's syndrome, SLE, polyarteritis nodosa, or Wegener's granulomatosis. Leukocytoclastic vasculitis may also arise secondary to drugs, usually antibiotics. Several terms, including hypersensitivity vasculitis, allergic vasculitis, or small-vessel necrotizing vasculitis, have been applied to these syndromes. The incidence is unknown, but the condition is fairly common, with no known gender or racial predilection.

Lesions of leukocytoclastic vasculitis usually appear in crops and evolve over several hours, from erythematous macules to palpable purpuric lesions 3–10 mm in diameter, most commonly in dependent areas. The center of the lesion becomes hemorrhagic. Individual lesions persist for less than a month and heal without scarring, yet often leave an area of post-inflammatory hyperpigmentation.

The histologic appearance is so characteristic that it has been given a specific name: leukocytoclastic vasculitis. Affected post-capillary venules are involved by a neutrophil-rich infiltrate, nuclear debris from degenerating neutrophils (leukocytoclasis), and fibrinoid necrosis. Direct immunofluorescence for immunoglobulin deposition is present in 60–80% of cases. IgA deposition is associated with Henoch-Schönlein purpura.

Laboratory findings may include elevated ESR, low serum complement levels, circulating cryoglobulins, and anemia. Despite the hemorrhagic nature of the lesions, there is no thrombocytopenia or coagulopathy.

The occurrence of leukocytoclastic vasculitis should lead one to search for an underlying cause. Screening tests for SLE (ANA), Wegener's granulomatosis (ANCA), viral hepatitis, and cryoglobulinemia should be performed.

Drug-induced leukocytoclastic vasculitis has been reported following administration of several types of medications. Antibiotics are the most frequent causative drugs, with penicillins accounting for most reports. Cutaneous vasculitis has also been reported in patients receiving allopurinol, sulfonamides, thiazide diuretics, β-blockers, or hydantoins. The pathologic appearance of drug-associated lesions may be leukocytoclastic, although mononuclear cell infiltration of the vessels has also been reported.

The prognosis of palpable purpura depends on the extent, as well as the underlying cause. If vasculitis is limited to the skin, the prognosis is good. Likewise, treatment depends on the extent and duration of involvement. For an initial eruption in a patient with no evidence of systemic involvement, symptomatic treatment, such as reduction of activity and leg elevation, may be sufficient. For recurrent lesions, colchicine has been advocated. Dapsone and antimalarial drugs also have been employed with variable success. The use of oral corticosteroid is reserved for resistant cases or those associated with underlying diseases that are known to respond to steroid medication.

The present patient had characteristic skin lesions with histopathologic features of a leukocytoclastic vasculitis. There was no evidence of underlying disease. He was treated by discontinuing the ampicillin. All lesions healed within 1 month, but residual post-inflammatory hyperpigmentation persisted.

Clinical Pearls

1. The clinical appearance of palpable purpura results from a characteristic vasculitis involving post-capillary dermal venules. The histology of this vasculitis is termed "leukocytoclastic," to describe the fragmented neutrophils characteristic of the lesions.

2. Leukocytoclastic vasculitis may be limited to the skin, or may be a cutaneous manifestation of an underlying illness such as SLE, Henoch-Schönlein purpura, polyarteritis nodosa, or Wegener's granulomatosis.

3. When IgA deposits are present on immunohistochemistry, the term Henoch-Schönlein purpura is applied.

4. Drug-induced leukocytoclastic vasculitis has been reported to be associated with several drug classes. Although penicillins account for the majority of case reports, sulfonamides, allopurinol, thiazide diuretics, and β-blockers have all been implicated.

REFERENCES

1. Callen JP. Colchicine is effective in controlling chronic cutaneous leukocytoclastic vasculitis. J Am Acad Dermatol 1985; 13:193–200.
2. Callen JP. Cutaneous vasculitis: Relationship to systemic disease and therapy. Curr Prob Dermatol 1993;37:187–192.
3. Jennette CJ, Milling DM, Falk RJ. Vasculitis affecting the skin: A review. Arch Dermatol 1994;130:899–906.
3. Roujeau JC, Stern RS. Severe adverse cutaneous reactions to drugs. N Engl J Med 1994;331:1272–1285.

INDEX

Page numbers in **boldface** indicate complete cases.